ADULT DAY CARE

The Johns Hopkins Series in Contemporary Medicine and Public Health

CONSULTING EDITORS

Martin D. Abeloff, M.D.

Samuel H. Boyer IV, M.D.

Gareth M. Green, M.D.

Richard T. Johnson, M.D.

Paul R. McHugh, M.D.

Edmond A. Murphy, M.D.

Edyth H. Schoenrich, M.D., M.P.H.

Jerry L. Spivak, M.D.

Barbara H. Starfield, M.D., M.P.H.

ALSO OF INTEREST IN THIS SERIES

William Halsey Barker, M.D., *Adding Life to Years: Organized Geriatrics Services in Great Britain and Implications for the United States*

Carl Eisdorfer, Ph.D., M.D., David A. Kessler, M.D., J.D., and Abby N. Spector, M.M.H.S., eds., *Caring for the Elderly: Reshaping Health Policy*

Nancy L. Mace, ed., *Dementia Care: Patient, Family, and Community*

Vincent Mor, Ph.D., David S. Greer, M.D., and Robert Kastenbaum, Ph.D., eds., *The Hospice Experiment*

Kevin Morgan, *Sleep and Aging: A Research-based Guide to Sleep in Later Life*

ADULT DAY CARE

FINDINGS FROM
A NATIONAL SURVEY

William G. Weissert
Jennifer M. Elston
Elise J. Bolda
William N. Zelman
Elizabeth Mutran
Anne B. Mangum

THE JOHNS HOPKINS UNIVERSITY PRESS

BALTIMORE · LONDON

The Johns Hopkins University Press, 701 West 40th Street, Baltimore, Maryland 21211
The Johns Hopkins Press Ltd., London

The paper used in this publication meets the minimum requirements of American
National Standard for Information Sciences—Permanence of Paper for Printed Library
Materials, ANSI Z39.48-1984.

Library of Congress Cataloging-in-Publication Data

Adult day care : findings from a national survey / William G. Weissert . . . [et al.].
p.   cm. — (The Johns Hopkins series in contemporary medicine and public health)
Includes bibliographical references.
ISBN 0-8018-4001-5 (alk. paper)
1. Day care centers for the aged—United States. I. Weissert, William G. II. Series.
[DNLM: 1. Day Care—in old age—United States. WT 29 AA1 A24] HV1455.2.U6A38
1990 362.6'3—dc20   DNLM/DLC   for Library of Congress   90-4112

*To the generous and caring staff members
of America's adult day care centers and
to their participants*

CONTENTS

PREFACE

THIS BOOK was based upon a national survey project conducted with the cooperation of the 60 adult day care centers, their staff, and their users, who participated in the study, the National Council on Aging's National Institute of Adult Day Care (NIAD), its steering committee and staff directors, Ms. Betty Ransom (former director) and Ms. Dorothy Howe (current director), the project's advisory committee, the generous support of the John A. Hartford Foundation, and the expert assistance of many outstanding researchers and practitioners.

Biostatistical expertise was provided by Professor Gary Koch, Associate Professor William Kalsbeek, and doctoral student Wendy Foran of The University of North Carolina's School of Public Health (UNCSPH) Biostatistics Department. Financial management analysis was directed by Associate Professor William Zelman, C.P.A., of UNCSPH Health Policy and Administration Department. Analysis of satisfaction data was conducted by Associate Professor Elizabeth Mutran of UNCSPH Health Behavior and Health Education Department. Description of the clinical aspects of adult day care and its participants was provided by Associate Professor Philip Sloane, M.D., of UNC School of Medicine Family Medicine Department. Assistance in economic issues was provided by Assistant Professor Thomas Rice of UNCSPH Health Policy and Administration Department. Econometric expertise was provided by Associate Professor Bryan Dowd of the Division of Health Services Research and Policy, School of Public Health at The University of Minnesota.

Project manager during data collection and data entry phases of the project, manager of the DayCare software development, and co-author of the utilization chapter was Ms. Elise Bolda, a doctoral student in the UNCSPH Department of Health Policy and Administration. Manager of the analytical and publication phases of the project and co-author of the models and regulation and financial chapters, was Ms. Jennifer Elston, now doctoral student in the Department of Health Services Organization and Policy in the School of Public Health at The University of Michigan. Editorial assistance in preparation of the entire manuscript was provided by Assistant Professor Ann Mangum of The University of North Carolina at Greensboro.

Mainframe computer programming was provided by Ms. Beth Beattie, now of Quintiles Inc., and Ms. Jane Darter, now of the Health Services

Research Center at The University of North Carolina. Fiscal data collection consultation was provided by Ms. Sandra Crawford Leak, research associate with Duke University Long Term Care Resource Program. Assistance in data analysis for the modeling chapter was provided by Ms. Cynthia Cready, former research associate with the UNCSPH Program on Aging.

The DayCare software was developed with the substantial assistance and expertise of Mr. Teiji Kimball, now microcomputing consultant at the North Carolina Memorial Hospital.

Students whose assistance was invaluable at various phases of the project include: Kristen Gooch and Ellen Pisarski, former students of the UNC Economics Department; Eleanor Blakely, of the UNC Curriculum in Public Policy Analysis; and Cindy Bateman, Wilma Case, Dawn Dalmas, Denise Levis, Catharine Wilson, and Shawn Zelmer, of the UNCSPH Department of Health Policy and Administration.

Special thanks is due to the members of the advisory committee composed of members of the NIAD's steering committee and two eminent home and community care researchers. They are (NIAD representatives) Dr. Ruth Von Behren, Ms. Sudie Goldston, Ms. Kay Larmer, and Ms. Dorothy Howe; Dr. Peter Kemper, Senior Research Manager at the National Center for Health Services Research, U.S. Department of Health and Human Services; and Dr. John Capitman, Director of Long Term Care, Bigel Institute for Health Policy, Heller School at Brandeis University.

Project instruments and data collection procedures were pilot tested at the Community Life Center in Durham, North Carolina, with the generous assistance and invaluable advice of Ms. Ann Johnson, Director of the Coordinating Council for Senior Citizens, her staff, and the center participants.

The original project idea was the brainchild of Ms. Ina Guzman of Washington, D.C., then project officer with the John A. Hartford Foundation. Evaluative feedback and direction were provided at interim points in the study by Ms. Laura Robbins, Project Officer, and Dr. Donna Regenstreif, Senior Program Officer for Health and Aging, of the John A. Hartford Foundation of New York City; Mr. Ronald Weismehl, Executive Vice President of the Council for Jewish Elderly of the Jewish Federation of Metropolitan Chicago, and Dr. Rosalie Kane, Professor, Division of Health Services Research and Policy, School of Public Health at The University of Minnesota and Editor of the *Gerontologist,* who served as outside reviewers for the John A. Hartford Foundation; and Dr. Thomas Wan, Professor of Health Services Administration at Virginia Commonwealth University, who served as an outside evaluator and project reviewer at the research team's request.

The entire manuscript and all correspondence associated with the project were typed by Ms. Carolyn Hammerle, now administrative assistant to the UNCSPH Curriculum in Public Health Nursing.

This crack team of national stature made this project a joy and success. The contributions of each person are gratefully acknowledged.

ADULT DAY CARE

ONE

MODELS OF ADULT DAY CARE

ADULT DAY CARE is one of a number of rapidly growing long-term care options that became available as health care expanded to encompass a variety of home- and community-based settings and services. Despite substantial evidence that day care usually is not a cost-effective substitute for nursing home care (Weissert et al., 1988), political support grows stronger each year (U.S. Congress, 1988).

Adult day care is of particular interest because it represents an entirely different setting for care, apart from the home, outpatient clinic, or institution. It was first systematically described in this country in the mid-1970s (Rathbone-McCuan, 1976; Weiler et al., 1976; Weissert, 1976, 1977, 1978; Weiler & Rathbone-McCuan, 1978). More recent surveys of national scope include those of Von Behren (1986), Mace & Rabins (1984), and Conrad et al. (1987).

The goal of our study was to describe this developing care modality after a decade of growth. (The National Institute of Adult Day Care celebrated its tenth anniversary in 1989.) Primary interest was directed toward day care users, the staffing and services offered by day care, and its costs, revenues, and client satisfaction. We were also interested to see whether day care centers serve different populations, and if so, how their services, staffing, costs, revenues, and participants' satisfaction differ. A conceptual model of day care center operations is depicted in Figure 1.1. It assumes that case mix determines staffing, services, utilization, operating costs, revenues, and satisfaction. This conceptual model was the basis for questionnaires and other methods used to acquire data for each domain depicted.

The National Survey

THE SAMPLE

Study data were obtained through a two-stage sample of day care centers and enrollees chosen through a national random sample of centers that had been in operation for at least one year as of July 1, 1985, and were

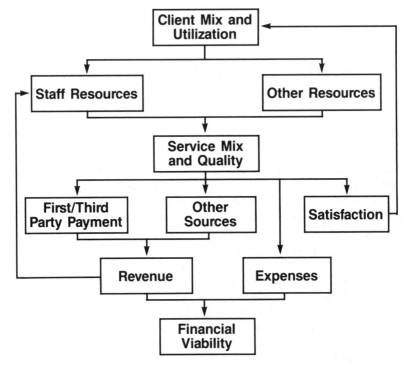

Figure 1.1. Conceptual model of adult day care.

located in Standard Metropolitan Statistical Areas (SMSAs) with 1980 populations of 80,000 or more. The first stage of selection was completed in two steps.

First, a systematic sample of 200 centers was drawn from a National Directory of Adult Day Care Centers (Department of Health and Human Services, 1980). To ensure a representative selection of centers, the list was ordered by three population size strata (populations greater than 1 million, between 250 thousand and 1 million, and between 80 thousand and less than 250 thousand), and by the ratio of nursing home beds to elderly population. Standard Metropolitan Statistical Areas with no centers in 1980 were attached to the ordered list of SMSAs with centers to ensure equal probability of their selection. From this list a simple random subsample of 28 centers was selected as the first-step sample.

Second, to allow inclusion of centers established since the directory was produced in 1980, its listings were updated within the selected SMSAs. Investigators identified new centers by telephoning all known centers, Area Agencies on Aging, state and local officials, and others likely to be familiar with the day care centers operating within a given SMSA. Newly identified centers were assigned appropriate probabilities for selection, and 35 more centers were drawn into the sample. This two-step sampling method resulted in selecting 63 centers for study. Sixty centers agreed to participate, representing a response rate of 95.2 percent among identified centers. Specific item response was at times lower, however, particularly for financial data that are traditionally difficult to obtain on such surveys, for example, the National Nursing Home Survey (National Center for Health Statistics, 1979).

In the second stage of sampling, a systematic random sample of at least eight participants per center was selected from enrollees who had attended within the preceding 30 days in each of the 60 centers. Participants were chosen by systematic sampling after a random start, the number drawn varying relative to each center's enrollment size. From these 529 participant record abstractions, a subsample of all participants who were present on the day(s) of the visit was interviewed.

A second subsample, this one of participant caregivers, was compiled from the sample of participants whose records had been selected for abstraction. That is, for all participants whose records were selected, staff members were asked to identify an at-home caregiver. If one was identified, the caregiver was interviewed by telephone. In total, 168 caregivers were interviewed.

Because selection probabilities differed among sample members in this design, a numerical weighting factor that accounted for this disproportionality and other common deficiencies encountered in survey practice (e.g., nonresponse) was computed for each center and its participants and caregivers. These weights were then used in all analyses.

DATA COLLECTION

Between July 1, 1985, and September 30, 1986, researchers made one- to two-day visits to each of the 60 participating centers. Questionnaires administered to center directors gathered information on center services, organizational relationships, affiliations, and staffing patterns. Facilities and equipment were inventoried and evaluated with a survey instrument that drew heavily on the Multiphasic Environmental Assessment Procedure (Moos & Lemke, 1984). Data on annual days of operation and participant use were collected from attendance logs. Revenue and expenditure data, including payroll information, were collected from existing financial reports and appropriate staff members.

Demographic, diagnostic, and functional data were collected from selected participants' records during each visit, and interviews were conducted with all those selected who were present on the day(s) of the visit. Interviews included the Short Portable Mental Status Questionnaire

(Pfeiffer, 1975) and items designed to assess levels of satisfaction with the day care center and its staff. The items on satisfaction were adapted and expanded from a variety of instruments reviewed by Kane and Kane (1981).

Telephone interviews were conducted with each identified caregiver to determine his or her relationship to the participant, the extent of help the caregiver provided to the participant, the reasons the participant and caregiver chose day care, and the caregiver's level of satisfaction with the day care center.

Results

MODELS OF ADULT DAY CARE

A study of adult day care in 1975 categorized day care centers into two broad types: health oriented and social services oriented (Weissert, 1976, 1977). That study showed that the two categories differed in participants, staffing, services, costs, and features likely to be associated with the center; in part, these differences resulted from the type of organization under whose auspices the center operated. One goal of our study was to determine if those two models, a single more inclusive model, or several models best describe adult day care as it exists at the end of the 1980s.

Because centers operating under different auspices are likely to contact clients with different needs, we hypothesized that centers of different auspices were likely to be serving different populations that could be distinguished by case-mix measures such as dependency in activities of daily living (ADL). We further hypothesized that these auspice/case-mix groupings would correlate with differences in other center characteristics, including staffing, services, costs, and revenues.

To begin the search for models, the relationship between auspices and case mix was examined. The percentage of participants at a center who were severely dependent (i.e., needing human help in toileting or eating), as well as the percentage independent in all ADLs (i.e., requiring no human assistance with bathing, dressing, toileting, transferring, continence, or eating), varied widely—from 0 to 100 percent—and, as expected, proved to be highly correlated with the auspices under which centers operated (Table 1.1).

Although the relationship of auspices to other case-mix measures (e.g., the percentage of participants who were independent in all activities of daily living, mobility dependent, diagnosed as having a mental illness, paid privately for their care, etc.) was explored with analysis of variance to analyze within- and between-group differences, dependency in toileting or eating proved to be most closely associated with auspices.

Table 1.1
The Relationship of Dependency and Auspices among Adult Day Care Centers

Auspice	Percentage needing help with toileting/eating[a]		Percentage ADL independent[b]	
	Mean	Range	Mean	Range
Mental health	5.4	0.0–12.5	85.7	75.0–100.0
Housing authority	8.3	0.0–25.0	53.8	12.5–87.5
Senior program	12.1	0.0–50.0	54.2	25.0–100.0
Other social service	21.0	0.0–54.5	53.8	25.0–90.0
Municipal	21.2	12.5–30.0	25.0	0.0–50.0
Hospital	23.1	0.0–87.5	62.5	0.0–87.5
Cerebral palsy	25.0	—	62.5	—
Freestanding	31.8	0.0–53.8	35.6	0.0–100.0
Veteran	33.3	—	22.2	—
Nursing home	44.7	14.3–100.0	23.1	0.0–71.4
Rehabilitation hospital	54.8	40.0–66.7	8.5	0.0–25.0
Blind	55.6	—	0.0	—

Note: n = 522 participants; n = 59 centers.
[a]Person receives human assistance with toileting or eating.
[b]Person receives no human assistance with bathing, dressing, toileting, transferring, continence, or eating (ADL, activity of daily living).

For the case-mix analysis, special purpose centers (i.e., centers serving only the veterans, those with cerebral palsy, and mentally ill and blind individuals) were eliminated as each of these centers served a unique clientele and was clearly different from one another and from remaining centers. Then, using the percentage of participants who were severely dependent as the criterion variable, an overall analysis of variance showed the existence of distinct differences (p = .015) among the eight auspice-affiliated centers (i.e., freestanding, nursing home, hospital, rehabilitation hospital, senior program, municipal, housing authority, and other social service) (Table 1.2). Assessment of the pairwise comparisons found that (1) statistically significant differences occur between nursing home– or rehabilitation hospital–affiliated programs and the other 6 auspices in 8 of 12 possible individual comparisons; (2) no significant differences exist between nursing home– and rehabilitation hospital–affiliated centers (p = .46); and (3) for centers not affiliated with a nursing home or rehabilitation hospital, among the 15 pairwise comparisons none differ significantly (p > .05).

Given the findings, the eight affiliations were combined into two aus-

Table 1.2
Least Squares Means Analysis of Adult Day Care Models

PROB > |T| H : LSMEANS (I) = LSMEANS (J)

Auspice	Percentage severely dependent	Rehabilitation hospital	Nursing home	Freestanding	General hospital	Municipal	Social service	Senior program	Housing authority
Rehabilitation hospital	54.8	—	—	—	—	—	—	—	—
Nursing home	44.7	.46	—	—	—	—	—	—	—
Freestanding	31.8	.11	.17	—	—	—	—	—	—
General hospital	23.1	.04	.04	.42	—	—	—	—	—
Municipal	21.3	.12	.20	.58	.92	—	—	—	—
Social service	21.0	.02	.02	.31	.85	.99	—	—	—
Senior program	13.1	.01	.01	.14	.44	.68	.54	—	—
Housing authority	8.3	.01	.00	.06	.25	.52	.33	.74	—

Note: n = 480 participants; n = 53 centers; dependent variable, percentage of participants receiving human assistance with toileting or eating.

pice/case-mix models: nursing home/rehabilitation and general hospital/ social service agency. Goodness of fit of the two-model categorization of auspices and case mix was evaluated by observing that the change in variability in case mix explained by auspices for the two-group analysis relative to the eight-group analyses was nonsignificant ($p > .25$) for the criterion variable, severe physical dependency. The two-model categorization explained 74.3 percent of the case-mix variation found within the eight auspice-affiliated centers.

The small lack of compatibility with the two-model categorization is primarily the result of some ambiguity in the classification of freestanding centers, for which severe physical dependency levels were somewhat below those for nursing home and rehabilitation hospital centers and somewhat above those for the other five affiliations. For the purposes of this study, freestanding affiliations are categorized as belonging to Model II (general hospital/social service agency), because other program characteristics support this assignment. Figure 1.2 illustrates the three models and their prevalence within the sample, and Figure 1.3 illustrates the prevalence of participants among the three models. Although exceptions exist, in general centers affiliated with senior centers, general hospitals, and other social service agencies tend to have fewer severely dependent and more independent participants than those affiliated with nursing homes and rehabilitation hospitals, which tend to have many severely dependent and few independent participants.

These findings suggest that day care is not one single entity, but as with hospitals and nursing homes is best characterized by subgroups of centers that are similar to each other and different from those of other subgroups. Which persons use a center appears to be influenced by the type of clien-

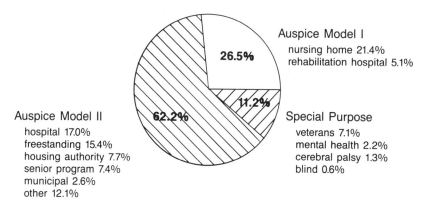

Auspice Model I
nursing home 21.4%
rehabilitation hospital 5.1%

Auspice Model II
hospital 17.0%
freestanding 15.4%
housing authority 7.7%
senior program 7.4%
municipal 2.6%
other 12.1%

Special Purpose
veterans 7.1%
mental health 2.2%
cerebral palsy 1.3%
blind 0.6%

Figure 1.2. Three models of day care: percentage of centers ($n = 529$ participants; $n = 59$ centers).

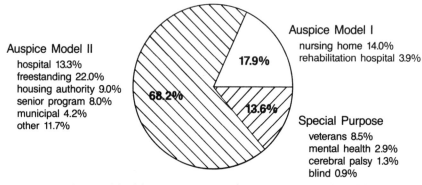

Auspice Model II
hospital 13.3%
freestanding 22.0%
housing authority 9.0%
senior program 8.0%
municipal 4.2%
other 11.7%

Auspice Model I
nursing home 14.0%
rehabilitation hospital 3.9%

Special Purpose
veterans 8.5%
mental health 2.9%
cerebral palsy 1.3%
blind 0.9%

Figure 1.3. Three models of day care: percentage of participants (n = 529 participants; n = 59 centers).

tele associated with the agency that spawned the day care center. Analytically, auspices may be considered as an exogenous variable to the model that was shown in Figure 1.1.

The remainder of this chapter presents descriptive statistics on a wide variety of day care center characteristics, and compares and contrasts differences among the three models. Model differences among categorical variables were evaluated for statistical significance using chi-square (χ^2) tests for overall and pairwise comparisons, with continuity corrections being used for the latter. For continuous variables, analyses of variance methods were used as described previously. Because the expenditure and revenue data had skewed distributions, analysis-of-variance methods were applied to their ranks to approximate a nonparametric analysis. In all analyses, weights based on the sampling design were taken into account, and thus findings apply to the survey population. Other adjustments for the structure of the sampling design were not applied because the methods described here were considered to yield reasonable estimates of variability and test statistics.

Special Purpose centers each serve a homogenous population and are heterogeneous as a group; thus, there is no typical special purpose center, and means and other summary statistics therefore are less useful in describing them than they are for characterizing Model I and Model II centers. This is particularly problematic when describing typical participants of the three models.

PARTICIPANT CHARACTERISTICS

Participant descriptive data overall and for each of the three models are shown in Table 1.3. For comparison, residents of nursing homes, as well as individuals living in the community, are shown. For clarity of presenta-

Table 1.3
A Comparison of Elderly Adult Day Care Participants with Elderly Nursing Home Residents and Dependent Elderly Persons in the Community

	Average age	Over age 84	Female	White	Married	Living alone	Mental disorder[a]	ADL dependencies None[b]	ADL dependencies Toileting/eating	ADL dependencies Average number	IADL dependencies None[c]	IADL dependencies Average number	Prior inpatient use Nursing home (ever)	Prior inpatient use Mental hospital (ever)	Prior inpatient use Hospital (in past 12 months)
Community[d]	73.4	7.2%	59.2%	90.5%	55.1%	31.8%	3.4%	92.6%	2.6%	0.2	77.3%	0.3	2.0%	NA	19.5%
Nursing home[e]	83.0	45.3	74.7	93.1	13.0	NA	48.3	7.9	65.5	3.9	NA	NA	NA	NA	NA
Adult day care	77.7	19.6	63.8	73.3	28.9	27.6	37.9	44.7	27.7	1.5	38.5	1.1	8.6	12.9%	32.7
Auspice Model I	79.2	29.6+	64.2	95.0+	39.5	19.9	24.6*	24.7+	42.7+	2.3*	36.8	-.9	17.8+	8.0	25.1
Auspice Model II	77.4	14.5+	70.5	64.9+	19.7*	31.8	41.2	54.9+	21.7+	1.2	40.5	1.1	5.0+	15.9	35.0
Special Purpose	75.8	22.5	25.7*	62.8	53.7	23.8	52.9	38.5	23.5	1.1	32.1	1.4	3.8	9.6	39.0

Note: Includes only individuals over the age of 64; $n = 401$.

[a]Includes ICD-9 codes 290–319.

[b]Person receives no human assistance with bathing, dressing, toileting, transferring, continence, or eating.

[c]Person receives no human assistance with mobility, meal preparation, money management, shopping, or administering medication.

[d]*Source:* 1984 National Health Interview Survey's Supplement on Aging.

[e]*Source:* 1985 National Nursing Home Survey.

*Indicates that value is significantly ($p < .05$) different from other two day care model values.

+Indicates that pairwise difference is significant ($p < .05$).

tion, nonelderly persons (those under age 65) are excluded from all populations shown in the table. The percentage of nonelderly participants was relatively low in all centers, averaging 18 percent. (Descriptive data for the nonelderly population are included in Appendix Table A.1 on page 117.)

Among elderly participants the average age was almost 78 years, with just under 20 percent being older than 84 years. Most participants were white, unmarried females who did not live alone. In addition, more than half of all participants were functionally dependent and almost 40 percent suffered from a mental disorder. Almost one-third of all participants had been hospitalized during the past year, while less than one-fifth had spent time in a nursing home in the past year.

In comparing differences in participant characteristics among the three models, the percentage of nonelderly participants ranged from a high of 31 percent of the population in Special Purpose centers to a low of 15 percent in Auspice Model II centers; this difference was not statistically different among the models.

Differences among elderly participants of the three models appear to validate the usefulness of the groupings. Each model served distinct populations. Elderly participants in Auspice Model I (centers affiliated with nursing homes and rehabilitation hospitals) were the most physically dependent, manifesting more of the characteristics associated with nursing home institutionalization than elderly participants of either of the other two models. They were significantly more likely than Model II participants to have been in a nursing home, to be over 85, to be married, and to be white, and were significantly more likely than Special Purpose participants to be female. They were also dependent in significantly more functions than participants in the other two categories. A more detailed profile of ADL dependency by Auspice Model is presented in Table 1.4.

Table 1.4
The Prevalence of Dependency in Activities of Daily Living by Model

	Percent dependent[a]					
	Eat	Transfer	Toilet	Dress	Bath	None
Overall average	16.4	12.9	3.4	11.9	9.9	45.9
Auspice Model I	33.2	14.3	4.1	12.4	13.4	22.4
Auspice Model II	12.4	11.1	3.8	11.0	7.7	55.3
Special Purpose	14.2	19.9	0.0	15.8	16.3	30.4

[a]Individuals are classified into their most severe level of dependency.

With respect to mental disorders, Model I participants were significantly less likely to have such a diagnosis compared to Model II and Special Purpose center participants. Auspice Model II participants, in comparison to Model I, were more likely to serve a racially minority population, probably reflecting the predominately social service agency affiliations of Model II.

Four case studies are listed below that illustrate the diversity of social and health-related needs manifested by clients receiving adult day care in the different models.

AUSPICE MODEL I

Case 1: An elderly widower with a prior hip fracture lives alone. His children visit every two weeks, but are not involved in his day-to-day care. Alert and oriented, he walks with an unsteady gait secondary to proximal muscle weakness that developed after his hip fracture. Services provided by adult day care include monitoring his seizure medications, helping him obtain a hearing aid, providing two meals per day, getting him out of the house, providing a sympathetic ear, and giving him a bath (because of mobility problems, he is afraid to bathe at home).

Case 2: An 88-year-old Russian immigrant has diabetes and mild dementia, complicated by language problems and moderate hearing loss. He lives with his psychiatrically disabled son and his grandson, who has ulcerative colitis. Neither the son nor the grandson can adequately care for him or reliably administer his daily insulin. When not at adult day care, he receives insulin injections daily from a visiting nurse. For less than the daily cost of that nurse visit, he receives insulin, has the remainder of his daily medication placed in envelopes, is fed two meals, and is encouraged to walk. The center also sets up his physician appointments and arranges transportation to them, has helped him obtain glasses, and writes letters for him.

AUSPICE MODEL II

Case 3: A 68-year-old woman has osteoarthritis of the spine and hips and weighs 278 pounds. She uses a walker or cane to ambulate, but can perform all activities of daily living. She lives alone in a high-rise apartment and does her own housework, but tires easily. Hearing, communication, and mental status are good. She identifies the major benefits of adult day care as participating in discussion and exercise groups and socializing with other people.

SPECIAL PURPOSE CENTER

Case 4: A 70-year-old white man has multiple injuries sustained during World War II, including the loss of an eye and a more recent history of stroke, which has resulted in difficulties with ambulation and communication. He is married, lives with his wife, and has no children. He frequently becomes confused and is often forgetful, thus requiring supervision. He also requires assistance with personal care. While at the center he receives speech therapy, case management, and has access to a physician on a weekly basis for his routine health care needs.

While some day care participants appear to share many characteristics with nursing home residents, day care participants differed sharply from typical nursing home residents both collectively and in each of the three models. In general, nursing home residents were about four years older and more than twice as likely to be over age 85 than day care participants, and they were more likely to be unmarried, functionally dependent, and dependent in more activities of daily living than day care participants.

As a group, elderly participants of Model II centers were most like elderly individuals living in the community (see Table 1.3). (Of course, elderly day care participants themselves constitute a subgroup—albeit a small one—of elderly living in the community.) Compared to community residents, a slightly lower proportion of Model II participants were white, female, or married. More day care participants than community residents had spent time in a mental hospital and were dependent in an instrumental activity of daily living (IADL).

CENTER PURPOSES

Although center directors were often aware that day care does not usually serve as a substitute for nursing home care, printed center materials and questionnaire responses indicated that one of the many purposes of their center was to delay or avoid institutionalization. Directors also emphasized social interaction and recreation, rehabilitative training/skill building, or health monitoring and maintenance. Caregiver respite also was a goal of some centers, as was assistance with transitional periods (i.e., between hospital or nursing home and home).

Directors of Special Purpose centers, none of whom saw their centers as providing aid for transitional periods, were significantly more likely than Model II directors to think of their centers as providing respite to the informal caregiver. Model II directors were significantly more likely to list health maintenance and monitoring as a primary purpose than Model I directors. Although this seems counterintuitive given the clientele each model is serving, it may simply reflect the likelihood that day care is no different from other industries inasmuch as stated goals often are inconsistent with operations. Model II programs may experience a greater need to emphasize the health care aspect of their services in an effort to secure certification for funding from sources such as Medicaid, and thus they may not apply as rigorous a definition to health maintenance and monitoring as do Model I centers.

ACTIVITIES

Information gathered from daily program schedules and the site-visit team's observations suggested that what centers most often do, at least as a minimum, is offer individuals a place to go during the day where social interaction, exercise, and a hot noontime meal are available and where nursing observation and supervision are provided.

A typical center's daily activity schedule is given here:

8:30–9:15 A.M	Early arrivals/coffee/visiting
9:15–9:45 A.M.	More arrivals/reality orientation/current events
9:45–10:45 A.M.	Late arrivals/exercise/therapies/health monitoring
10:45–11:45 A.M.	Arts and crafts
11:45–1:00 P.M.	Lunch/rest
1:00–2:00 P.M.	Visiting speaker/musician/movie
2:00–3:00 P.M.	Games/individual activities/early departures
3:00–3:30 P.M.	Snack/departure

Centers were open, on average, almost 8.5 hours per day; the range was from 4 to 11 hours. Centers opened as early as 7:00 A.M. and closed between 12:30 and 6:00 P.M., but most scheduled activities occurred between 9:00 A.M and 3:00 P.M., creating a structured, 6-hour day.

SERVICES

In addition to the foregoing activities, many centers provide varying degrees of case management, health assessment, nutrition education, therapeutic diets, transportation services, and counseling. Less frequently offered services include physical, occupational or speech therapies, physician services, breakfast, and dental services.

Table 1.5 illustrates the variety of health and social services offered by day care centers. Services may be provided directly by program staff, by contract, or through referral to other providers. They may be offered daily, weekly, monthly, or as needs of participants dictate.

In general, Model I centers were more likely than the others to provide

Table 1.5
The Services, Staffing Ratios, and Facility Characteristics of Three Models of
Adult Day Care

Center characteristics	Overall	Auspice Model I	Auspice Model II	Special Purpose
Health Services				
Nursing[a]	79%	96%	86%	9%*
Health assessment[c]	69	74	65	79
Therapeutic diets[a]	66	100*	51	33
Physical therapy[b]	42	61+	40	0+
Bathing[b]	30	59+	20+	0
Occupational therapy[b]	26	48	18	0
Physician[c]	21	26	21	9
Speech therapy[b]	19	43+	7+	12
Drug consultation[c]	15	26	10	0
Dentist[c]	12	21	10	0
Social/Supportive Services				
Case management[c]	71%	53%	79%	79%
Nutrition education[c]	68	58	87+	21+
Transportation to/from[a]	63	52	84+	12+
Professional counsel[c]	60	67	70+	9+
Church[c]	58	71+	64	9+
Music[c]	56	26+	70+	76
Hair care[c]	44	80*	32	9
Breakfast[a]	32	79*	12	9
Other transportation[c]	21	6	30	21
Meals-to-home[a]	10	22	5	0
Staff-to-Participant Ratios[d]				
All	.34:1	.46:1+	.23:1+	NA
Program director	.05:1	.07:1+	.04:1+	NA
LPN and RN	.04:1	.05:1	.03:1	NA
Activity aides	.04:1	.02:1+	.06:1+	NA
Nurses' aides	.03:1	.07:1+	.00:1+	NA
Social worker	.01:1	.02:1+	.01:1+	NA
Facility				
Median square feet/participant	136.0	155.8	123.0	217.0*
Meet 504 standards	88.2%	100.0%	94.3%	33.2%*

continued

Table 1.5 *continued*

Center characteristics	Overall	Auspice Model I	Auspice Model II	Special Purpose
Facility				
Annual fire inspection	83.3	80.9	82.2	91.0
Outside area	68.2	100.0*	62.3	28.4
Annual health inspection	51.6	78.1	53.4	0.0*
Special bathing facilities	49.5	86.7+	29.2+	46.2

aFor service to be counted as available, it must be provided either by program staff or on contract at least daily.

bFor service to be counted as available, it must be provided either by program staff or on contract at least weekly.

cFor service to be counted as available, it must be provided either by program staff or on contract at least monthly.

dRatios exclude nonpaid and in-kind staff.

*Indicates that value is significantly ($p < .05$) different from other two day care model values.

+Indicates that pairwise difference is significant ($p < .05$).

therapeutic and other health-related services, while Model II centers were more likely to provide social and supportive services, although many offered a variety of health care services. All Model I centers in our sample offered therapeutic diets, a capability associated with their inpatient facility affiliation.

Model II centers were significantly more likely than Special Purpose centers to provide daily transportation to and from the center as a direct service. The typical mode of transportation was a van equipped with a wheelchair lift. Van drivers assisted participants with activities such as dressing, leaving their residence (which could include carrying wheelchair-confined individuals downstairs), and boarding the van.

On the other hand, Model I centers were much more likely to offer transportation to medical appointments, shopping, or bill-paying on a monthly basis or more frequently (see Table 1.5).

No significant differences existed among models in the provision of case management services. (Case management, a loosely defined term in the long-term care lexicon, may include some or all the following: health assessment, care planning, arranging for services, monitoring services, and periodic reassessment.)

STAFFING

Typical center staffing included a director, often trained as a nurse or social worker, and an assistant plus some or all of the following: recreation/activity and nursing aides; nurses and therapists; custodial workers and van drivers; case managers and social workers; and administrative personnel and office staff.

Most staff members were paid employees. Consultant agreements tended to be for the services of a physician or therapist, while in-kind staffing was usually for fiscal manager or bookkeeping services.

While no significant differences were found among the models in the staff mix, Model I centers had significantly higher staff-to-participant ratios than Model II centers (see Table 1.5). (Staffing data for Special Purpose centers are not reported because few of such centers reported that information.)

FACILITIES

A large majority of day care centers were housed in multipurpose facilities. Common among those purposes were nursing homes, senior centers, and churches. Although some centers were affiliated with hospitals, none was physically located in the hospital building. As would be expected, Auspice Model I centers were most likely to be housed in a nursing home.

Interior space ranged from one large room to multiple rooms and office space, with a median of 136 square feet per participant (see Table 1.5). Centers were usually housed in facilities with an outside area available for participant use. Special Purpose centers on average had significantly more space per participant than those of the other two categories, but they were significantly less likely to meet Section 504 standards for handicapped access or to be inspected annually by a health department.

EQUIPMENT

Centers often had access to a wide variety of equipment. Most common among these were arts and crafts supplies, refrigerators, audiovisual equipment (record players, tape recorders, projectors, radios, television sets), pianos, library books, and wheelchairs. Most centers also had reality orientation materials, horticultural materials, video equipment, sewing machines, exercise equipment, quilting and weaving supplies, musical instruments, and beds or cots.

Model I centers were significantly more likely to have physical therapy, bathing, and hair care facilities, consistent with their inpatient facility locations. Otherwise, little difference was found among the three models with regard to equipment availability.

The average daily census at centers varied from a low of 5.6 to a high of 42.2, averaging just under 20 participants a day. The average daily census of Model II centers (23) was significantly higher than that of either Model I (15) or Special Purpose centers (16). The average elderly participant attended 3.4 days per week and just under 6 hours per day. Extremes ranged from 1 to 6 days per week. Attendance was most frequent in Model II centers (3.7 days per week), slightly less frequent in Model I centers (3.1 days per week), and least frequent in Special Purpose centers (2.5 days per week). (A more detailed analysis of utilization patterns is provided in Chapter 2.)

Adult day care received high marks as both participants and caregivers expressed high levels of satisfaction. Satisfaction of caregivers and elderly participants with the overall program ran particularly high, with 82.2 percent of the elderly participants and 92.3 percent of their caregivers reporting the highest level of satisfaction. Even more elderly participants said that they were completely satisfied with their transportation to and from the center (96 percent), the amount of attention they received from the staff (91 percent), and the program hours (91 percent). There was a little more disagreement about quality of food (79 percent), noise level (74 percent), center temperature (73 percent), and crowdedness (69 percent) No difference in levels of participant satisfaction was detected between the two Auspice models. (The small sample size for Special Purpose centers precludes discussion of differences between it and the Auspice models.) (A more detailed analysis of participant and caregiver satisfaction is provided in Chapter 3.)

A profile of a typical center constructed from median data shows revenues of approximately $140,000 and expenses that are slightly higher. Most of the revenues came from federal sources, with Medicaid being the largest single source. Auspice Model I centers, many of which were associated with nursing homes or had religious affiliations, were considerably less reliant upon federal funding than were Model II centers (Table 1.6).

Table 1.6
Median Percentage of Total Revenue Received by Source and Model

	Revenue source		
	Federal	Self-pay	Other nongovernment
Overall median	51.2	0.0	13.4
Auspice Model I	26.5 +	18.5	22.7
Auspice Model II	67.3 +	0.0	4.1

+ Indicates that pairwise difference is significant ($p < .05$).

Day care is a labor-intensive industry; labor accounted for more than 50 percent of reported costs. The other three major expense categories were transportation, facility, and food. On average, these four categories accounted for almost 85 percent of the total expenses incurred by a center, although the range was from slightly less than 60 to 100 percent. For all centers, about 10 percent of expenses were in kind, although Model I centers in general reported only a negligible amount of in-kind expenses. Finally, although across all centers there was a slightly negative median bottom line, the median margin of Model I centers was a positive 6 percent.

Reported total daily participant expenses ranged from a low of $9.88 to a high of $105.62. The median expense per participant day was $29.51. Expenses of most centers (80 percent) ranged from approximately $13 to $52; half were between $23 and $36. Table 1.7 reports median annual expenses by category and model. Note that Model I centers incurred labor, facility, and food costs per participant day that were significantly higher than those of Model II.

A detailed description of the financial data collected, the necessary adjustments made to the data, and an in-depth discussion of the findings are provided in Chapter 5.

Conclusions

Our primary interest was to describe the characteristics of day care centers and their participants. We found that centers provide, at a minimum, social interaction, exercise, and a hot noontime meal. In addition, nursing observation and supervision, case management, health assessment, nutrition education, therapeutic diets, transportation services, and counseling are likely to be available.

Centers serve an average of almost 20 participants per day. Many cen-

Table 1.7
Median Expenses per Participant Day by Model

Expense	Overall median	Auspice Model I	Auspice Model II
Total cost/participant day	$29.41	$31.20	$29.17
Labor cost/participant day	14.62	22.77 +	14.24 +
Transportation cost/participant day	3.31	4.03	3.05
Facility cost/participant day	2.66	5.15 +	2.62 +
Food cost/participant day	2.37	2.47 +	1.81 +

+ Indicates that pairwise difference is significant ($p < .05$).

ters rely heavily on the assistance of federal funds, most often from Medicaid, and some centers receive substantial funds from private philanthropic sources.

Findings indicate that although most day care participants are functionally dependent elderly, white, unmarried females, almost one-third of whom suffer from a mental disorder, participants do not closely resemble nursing home residents: they are younger, more likely to be married, less dependent, and less frequently mentally impaired.

We also hypothesized that center populations would be determined in part by the type of agency with which they were affiliated. Results indicate that day care centers currently operating in the United States can be categorized into three distinctive types:

Auspice Model I centers were defined as those affiliated with a nursing home or rehabilitation hospital. They typically provide services to a physically dependent, older, white population, most of whom do not suffer a mental disorder. Nursing, therapies, therapeutic diets, and other health and social services were provided by a complement of staff approaching one staff member for every two participants. Transportation to and from other services, especially health care services, is often available. Revenues come more from philanthropic and self-pay sources than governmental sources.

Auspice Model II centers were defined as those affiliated with a general hospital or a social services or housing agency. They typically serve a predominately unmarried, female population that frequently is a racial minority; most are under 85, typically are not dependent or only minimally dependent in activities of daily living, but more than 40 percent may be suffering a mental disorder. Services they receive include case management, nutrition education, professional counseling, transportation to and from the center, and frequently health assessment. Revenues come heavily from governmental sources, particularly Medicaid.

Special Purpose centers were defined as those that serve a single type of clientele each, such as the blind, the mentally ill, or service veterans. Their participant populations are as a result homogeneous within a center, but heterogeneous among centers within the same model. Although averages were presented as a point of reference for these centers, their within-group variability makes such summary statistics less meaningful than those for Models I and II.

Although these models are based on the correlation between auspices and case mix, they also were found to correlate with staffing, services, facilities, and revenues, presumably reflecting population needs as well as organizational resources.

The importance of these model distinctions is in part a function of the type of question being asked. While the distinctions are not important from a total daily cost perspective, they do capture important differences in the structure of daily costs. Likewise, the models suggest differences in how centers would be affected by changes in Medicaid reimbursement policy or the availability of block grant funds. In addition, the models would be important if one were asking this question: "Can day care centers serve a population which needs special diets, therapeutic services, or a high staff-to-participant ratio." The answer, on the basis of data presented here, would be "yes" for centers associated with nursing homes and rehabilitation hospitals, but only "perhaps" for other centers. Finally, for an agency thinking about developing a day care center, the models—while not deterministic—presage the type of clientele likely to be attracted and the types and levels of staffing and services typically associated with that particular auspice and case mix.

One overall change is worth noting. During the decade since the last study of this type, the Model II type of day care has broadened its mission to take on more health-related activities and health care staff (possibly influenced by state certification and licensure requirements). It is serving a population more likely to suffer mental disorders than was typical of the day care population studied 10 years ago in a small number of centers. Another change is the addition of Special Purpose centers. These centers, run by agencies that exist to serve a specialized client population, did not exist a decade ago. They add a new dimension to the variety of day care settings, and by definition make it true that affiliation of a day care center influences—often through eligibility criteria (e.g., only veterans)—its client mix.

One dimension of day care, cost, did not change much over the decade.

Irrespective of model, day care is a financial bargain. While a visit from a home health nurse may cost more than $40 and may last less than an hour, and a four-hour visit from a homemaker may cost more than $25, a visit to a day care center typically costs only about $30 a day and lasts nearly six hours, plus an hour of transportation. The day care center offers periodic health-assessment and case-management services, a daily meal, and interaction with other human beings—some are friends, others are professional caregivers and helpers. Even on days when participants are not attending, they or their personal caregiver can call the center for advice and assistance.

Finally, although previous research has shown that neither costs nor participant outcomes appear to be favorably altered by day care, and the current analysis shows (regardless of model) that most participants are at low risk of nursing home residency, participants and their caregivers are overwhelmingly satisfied with the care they receive. As such, day care centers are well positioned to meet the growing demand for programs offering respite care to informal caregivers, plus support to frail elderly individuals who would become eligible for expanded public subsidy if any of the congressional proposals previously mentioned is adopted.

TWO

FREQUENCY OF ATTENDANCE AMONG USERS OF ADULT DAY CARE

IN THIS CHAPTER, we discuss the reasons some participants attend day care 5 days per week while others attend less frequently.

Although several researchers have profiled correlates of acute and institutional long-term care use (Ward, 1977; Link et al., 1980; Scanlon, 1980; Wan & Odell, 1980; McCoy & Edwards, 1981; Roos & Shapiro, 1981; Branch & Jette, 1982; Brock & O'Sullivan, 1985; Hulka & Wheat, 1985; Shapiro & Tate, 1985; Cohen et al., 1986; Cafferata, 1987; Wingard et al., 1987; Mutran & Ferraro, 1988), multivariate analyses of elderly people's use of home- and community-based long-term care have been less frequently reported (Snider, 1980; Wan & Odell, 1980; Coulton & Frost, 1982; Krout, 1983; Soldo, 1983; Evashwick et al., 1984; Benjamin, 1986; Branch et al., 1988). These few reported studies suggest that many of the important correlates of acute and institutional utilization patterns are also important in describing use of home and community care.

Although many previous studies offer insight into the overall frequency of adult day care participation (Weissert, 1975, 1976, 1978; Kurland, 1982; Palmer, 1983; Hannan & O'Donnell, 1984; Mace & Rabins, 1984; Conrad et al., 1987), none is drawn from a representative national probability sample, and none provides empirical analyses of the participant and provider characteristics that influence utilization. This dearth of analysis based on national utilization data has led several researchers to call for such studies (Lloyd and Greenspan, 1985; Hawes et al., 1988).

This chapter focuses on the factors that appear to influence the frequency of day care participation, including six specific research questions regarding frequency of participation:

1. What difference, if any, does auspice make in attendance frequency? Does it serve as a filter interacting with and altering the likelihood of full-time attendance?
2. What individual characteristics distinguish full-time (five days/week) day care participants from part-time participants? Do these characteristics vary by auspice of the center attended?

3. How does public reimbursement policy affect full-time use? In particular, does Medicaid, as a payor of adult day care, act as a prudent buyer, rationing full-time use to only the most dependent Medicaid-eligible participants?
4. Does availability of transportation increase the likelihood of full-time use?
5. How do contextual factors such as county age structure, income, density, and competition from other day care centers affect full-time use?
6. How does percent of capacity used affect use? Do full centers ration full-time use to allow more participants access to services? Since most centers operate below capacity, are patterns likely to change if expanded public subsides increase demand, allowing more centers to operate closer to capacity?

Answers to these research questions should serve several purposes, including helping policy makers guage the impact of public subsidy on services delivered, helping providers estimate prospective clients' likely attendance patterns, and helping both providers and policy makers understand the adjustment to expected attendance patterns that must be made to account for competition and other contextual factors.

Data and Data Sources

Data came from three sources. (1) Participant characteristics and frequency of attendance came from the participant record; (2) center characteristics came from interviews with center directors; and (3) county characteristics came from the 1986 Area Resources File. Because the participant is the unit of analysis, variables measuring center and county characteristics were attached to the participant record.

Only data from the 45 centers categorized as either Auspice Model I or Auspice Model II from the national probability sample of 60 centers were considered in this analysis. (For a detailed description of data collection, the sample, methodology, and the auspice model categorization, see Chapter 1.) Special Purpose centers were excluded from utilization analyses because they typically serve narrowly defined participant pools (e.g., centers serving only persons who have a developmental disability, blindness, mental illness, etc.) and were too heterogeneous in their combined population to permit inclusion in this analysis.

The Model

Each participant's frequency of participation is defined on the basis of whether he or she attended full time (as many days per week as the center operated) or part time (fewer days per week than the day care center was open.) All centers in the analysis were open five days per week.

Attendance at adult day care (a dichotomous dependent variable coded 1 if full time and 0 if part time) was distributed relatively evenly within the sample: roughly 48 percent of all participants attended day care full time. The model used to estimate frequency of attendance hypothesizes that it is a function of participant characteristics, type of center attended, source of payment for care, availability of transportation, various contextual factors measured at the county level including competition from other day care providers in the county, and how close to capacity the center attended is operating.

The model includes 25 variables and 22 interaction terms. The latter were added to capture differences that could be attributed to the two types of center (Auspice Models I and II). It is possible that participants with similar characteristics would be more or less likely to attend day care full time, depending on the type of center they attend. These differences in attendance, if they existed, could represent the effects of differences between the two models in services, staffing, revenue sources, care philosophy, and other variables. Therefore, interaction terms for model and participant characteristics and model and county characteristics were added to the regression equation to estimate the modifying effects that the type of center might have on the attendance of participants.

The variables analyzed, the reasons they were included in the model, their expected positive or negative significance, and the findings are discussed here. The names and definitions of the variables are listed in Table 2.1.

Model Estimation Method

Individual variable means, logistic regression coefficients, and significance levels are presented in Table 2.2. The model was found to fit the data (model $\chi^2 = 1659.4$; df $= 47$; $p < .05$), and using the crude pseudo R^2 statistic (Aldrich & Nelson, 1986) explained approximately 40 percent of the variability in frequency of attendance. This model correctly classified 82 percent of the observations, with 15.5 percent false-positives (part-time users classified as full time) and 19.8 percent false-negatives (full-time users classified as part time).

Checks for multicolinearity among explanatory variables, nonlinearity, and effects of influential outliers were conducted and appropriate trans-

Table 2.1
Definition of the Variables

Dependent Variable	Coded 1 if:
Full-time	Participant attended daycare full-time
Independent Variables	Coded 1 if:
Age 85 +[a]	Participant was 85 or older
Male[a]	Participant was male
Married[a]	Participant was currently married
Prior Nursing Home Use[a]	Participant had been in a nursing home in the preceding 12 months
Toilet/Eating Dependent[a]	Participant was dependent in toileting, eating, or both
Mobility[a]	Participant had impaired mobility
Mental Illness[a]	Participant had mental illness other than dementia
Dementia	Participant had Alzheimer's or related dementia
Stroke[a]	Participant previously had a cerebral vascular accident
Cancer[a]	Participant previously had or currently has some type of neoplasm
Transport to/from Program	Transportation to and from center only
Comprehensive Transportation	Transportation to and from center and to other services
Density[a]	County population density above sample median
High Income[a]	County per capita income above sample median
High Income × Per Capita Income	High income county and per capita income
Private Pay[a]	Participant's daycare paid privately
Medicaid[a]	Participant's daycare paid by Medicaid
Medicaid × Toileting/ Eating Dependent[a]	Participant is dependent in these ADL and daycare paid for by Medicaid
Some Competition[a]	Number of daycare centers in county divided by county population age 65 and older is greater than 0 and less than the top tertile of distribution
High Competition[a]	Number of daycare centers in county (as above) is in the top tertile of sample distribution
Capacity Used[a]	Center average daily census divided by licensed daily capacity (or perceived capacity given current facilities and staffing if no licensed daily limit) is 90% or higher
Capacity × Density	High population density (above median) and top tertile of capacity used

continued

Table 2.1 *continued*

Independent Variables	Coded 1 if:
Northeast Region[a]	Center located in northeastern United States
Auspice Model I	Center attended is Auspice Model I (i.e., associated with a nursing home or rehabilitation facility and serving participants more likely to be dependent in toileting/eating than Model II participants)
County Age Structure[a]	Percent of persons age 65 and older in county age 85 or older
Per Capita Income[a]	County per capita income in 1982
Nursing Homes[a]	Number of nursing homes per person age 65 and older in county (logged)

[a]Terms interacted with Auspice Model I.

formations were undertaken when suggested by the values. For example, the positively skewed distribution of nursing homes per capita required log transformation.

The model was then reestimated using a weighted logistic regression package (Shah et al., 1984) developed specifically to account for complex sample design when calculating variances and significance levels. Results showed that design effects were small, and because they would not alter results, methods to adjust standard errors to correct for them were not used.

INTERPRETATION OF COEFFICIENTS

In general, the logistic regression coefficients reflect the percent change in the odds of full-time participation; a positive coefficient indicates an increased probability of full-time participation, and a negative coefficient indicates a decreased probability of full-time participation. Interpreting regression coefficients presented in Table 2.2 is somewhat complex, however, because of the interaction terms.

Specifically, the Auspice Model I variable, which has a large positive coefficient (see Table 2.2), cannot be interpreted straightforwardly. Because "auspice model" is interacted with several other variables, the effect of auspice model on full-time versus part-time use is dependent on the values of other variables with which auspice model is interacted. Therefore, the coefficient on Auspice Model I estimates the effect of auspice when all variables with which it is interacted are equal to zero—thus including, for example, the implausible event of a county with no elderly residents over 85. When all the interactive coefficients and the auspice

Table 2.2
Results of the Logistic Regression Analysis of Participant, Center, and Area Characteristics

Variable name	Mean	Coefficient	Level of signifi-cance
Dichotomous Variables			
Age 85 +	0.20302	2.06088	***
Auspice Model I × Age 85 +	0.10135	− 1.19848	***
Male	0.36919	0.20936	NS
Auspice Model I × Male	0.10988	− 2.46866	***
Married	0.27712	− 0.24540	NS
Auspice Model I × Married	0.09922	0.22379	NS
Prior Nursing Home Use	0.04342	1.43945	*
Auspice Model I × Prior Use	0.02481	− 3.33667	*
Toileting/eating dependent	0.25138	0.28594	NS
Auspice Model I × Toileting/Eating Dependent	0.09844	− 0.74785	NS
Mobility	0.37862	− 2.54689	***
Auspice Model I× Mobility	0.16982	1.51596	***
Mental illness	0.21443	1.08145	***
Auspice Model I × Mental Illness	0.05043	0.35094	NS
Dementia	0.25449	− 1.65128	***
Auspice Model I × Dementia	0.03500	1.42169	***
Stroke	0.19528	2.20736	***
Auspice Model I × Stroke	0.05311	− 3.27530	***
Cancer	0.02198	− 3.13746	*
Auspice Model I × Cancer	0.01057	16.24293	***
Transportation Available	0.80808	0.48432	NS
Auspice Model I × Transportation	0.13296	4.45399	NS
Density	0.61215	− 5.82581	***
Auspice Model I × Density	0.04128	− 2.99930	NS
High Income	0.63934	− 41.81831	***
Income Interaction	8848.44000	0.00381	***
Private Pay	0.44829	0.59685	***
Auspice Model I × Private Pay	0.19677	− 0.88878	*
Medicaid	0.21637	− 1.15266	***
Auspice Model I × Medicaid	0.03139	1.26239	*
Medicaid × Toileting/Eating	0.05570	5.55112	***
Auspice Model I × Medicaid × Toileting/Eating	0.01166	− 4.68388	***
Some Competition	0.92764	4.77062	***
Auspice Model I × Some Competition	0.23937	− 15.10589	*

continued

Table 2.2 *continued*

Variable name	Mean	Coefficient	Level of signifi-cance
Dichotomous Variables			
High Competition	0.49429	2.30533	***
Auspice Model I × High Competition	0.11083	17.37851	*
High Capacity Used	0.11366	−3.92410	***
Auspice Model I × High Capacity	0.03563	1.18111	NS
Capacity × Density	0.04121	2.02873	*
Northeast Region	0.52403	−7.26208	***
Auspice Model × Northeast	0.16168	0.72314	NS
Auspice Model I	0.28009	23.14339	***
Continuous Variables			
County Age Structure	8.62666	4.58993	***
Auspice Model I × County Age Structure	2.43266	−4.79228	***
Per Capita Income	12624.90000	−0.00281	***
Nursing Homes/1000 Elderly	−7.25125	−2.39969	***
Auspice Model I × Nursing Homes/El-derly	−2.11988	−2.16015	***
Intercept		−25.16151	

Note: ***, $p < .001$; *, $.001 < p < .1$; NS, not significant.

model coefficient are considered together (and percentage of elderly age 85 and older is within the true range), Auspice Model I participants are less likely to attend day care full time. This negative effect of Auspice Model I is counterintuitive given the large positive coefficient on the Auspice Model I variable.

In interpreting the coefficients of interaction terms for Auspice Model I and specific characteristics, the coefficient indicates the direction of the effect, such as improving or reducing the likelihood of being full time. For example, a positive coefficient for such an interaction by itself does not indicate that participants with the characteristic and who attend Auspice Model I centers are full-time users. Rather, because Auspice Model I has a negative effect on full-time attendance, a positive interaction coefficient simply would be interpreted as having "less" negative chances, or improved chances of being full time, though they may still be less likely to be full time than Auspice Model II users.

Results

For each of the characteristics discussed here, the reported influence of the characteristic being discussed assumes all other variables in the model are observed at the sample mean.

Question 1. What difference, if any, does auspice make in attendance frequency? Does it serve as a filter interacting with and altering the likelihood of full-time attendance?

Type of Center Attended Participants of Auspice Model I centers (affiliated with nursing homes and rehabilitation facilities) were significantly less likely to attend day care full time than were participants of Auspice Model II centers (affiliated with general hospitals/social service agencies).

Question 2. What individual characteristics distinguish full-time (five days per week) day care participants from part-time participants? Do these characteristics vary by type of center attended?

Age Previous research has shown that age is positively associated with increased use of health care services (Wan & Odell, 1980; Branch & Jette, 1982; Stoller, 1982; Evashwick et al., 1984; Brock & O'Sullivan, 1985; Cohen et al., 1986; Cafferata, 1987; Weissert & Cready, 1989). About 20 percent of the participants in the sample were 85 or older. As anticipated, older participants were more likely to be full-time day care attendants than younger participants. However, among participants attending Auspice Model I centers, the effect of being over 85 decreased the chances of a participant attending day care full time.

Gender Because men have been shown to be less frequent users of most health care services (Wan & Soifer, 1979; Coulton and Frost, 1982; Stoller, 1982; Evashwick et al., 1984; Shapiro and Tate, 1985)—with the exception of hospital services (Cafferata, 1987; Mutran & Ferraro, 1988)—it was anticipated that men would attend day care less frequently than women. Nearly 37 percent of the sample group of participants were male. The results indicated that in Auspice Model I centers men had a significantly reduced likelihood of being full time, although in general gender did not significantly influence frequency of attendance.

Marital Status In studies of both home- and community-based services, married persons have been found to have lower use rates than persons not currently married (Link et al., 1980; Branch and Jette, 1982; Soldo, 1983; Evashwick et al., 1984; Cohen et al., 1986; Weissert & Cready, 1989). In these cases, being married appears to imply social support and less dependence on others for nonacute care. Because approximately one-quarter of informal caregivers are employed, however, another reason that married participants might attend day care less frequently might be that the unmarried participants cared for by working caregivers are less able to rely on their social support system and therefore require more help from formal care.

In light of these expectations, the effect of being married—the status of about one-quarter of all participants—was anticipated to be negatively associated with full-time day care attendance. Results, however, showed that although the sign was negative as anticipated, marital status was not significantly related to frequency of attendance among day care users.

Prior Use Although prior use of health care services has been shown to increase utilization of hospital and nursing home services (Roos & Shapiro, 1981; Branch & Jette, 1982; Coulton & Frost, 1982; Evashwick et al., 1984; Shapiro & Tate, 1985; Branch et al., 1988; Mutran & Ferraro, 1988), little conclusive evidence about the effect of prior use of home- and community-based service has been reported.

Only 4 percent of all participants had been in a nursing home during the previous year. For them, a positive association between prior use of nursing homes and frequency of attendance was hypothesized on the basis of the nursing home and hospital use literature. Our results showed that a history of nursing home use did significantly increase the likelihood of full-time attendance, although prior nursing home placements had a negative influence on the chances of full-time attendance by Auspice Model I participants. This center effect may be caused by differences in the recency of prior use, in that more recent nursing home use (among Auspice Model I participants) may be associated with reduced stamina. Data on how recently participants had stayed in nursing homes were not available for more in-depth analyses.

Functional Dependency Higher levels of participant functional dependency were expected to be positively associated with full-time attendance, because previous research has shown that more dependent persons in both institutional and home- and community-based long-term care settings use health services more often (Branch & Jette, 1982; Soldo, 1983; Evashwick et al., 1984; Shapiro and Tate, 1985; Branch et al., 1988; Weissert and Cready, 1989). Among persons with dependencies in activities of daily living, those most dependent (i.e., eating, toileting) were expected to be more likely to use services full time. Participant dependency was also expected to be modified by the type of center attended and the source of payment for care.

Approximately one-quarter of all participants were reported to need some assistance with using the toilet or eating. Conversely, nearly half of all day care users were independent in activities of daily living. The effect of toileting/eating dependency on frequency of participation (comparing more and less dependent participants), although positive, was not significant. Similarly, no significant differences were found between models in frequency of attendance by participants with functional dependencies. These nonsignificant findings suggest that full-time versus part-time attendance was not strongly conditioned on dependency level (except among individuals subject to Medicaid's utilization control efforts, as discussed later in this chapter).

Mobility Because higher levels of dependency were expected to be associated with full-time attendance, participants with mobility impairments (controlling for functional dependencies) were expected to attend less often. No differences from center type were expected.

Slightly more than 35 percent of the day care users studied had some level of mobility impairment; fewer than 5 percent were confined to wheelchairs. In general, having impaired mobility was significantly related to less frequent attendance, and, comparing the two models, being mobility impaired and attending an Auspice Model I center further reduced the likelihood of attending day care full time.

Mental Illness/Cognitive Impairment Participants diagnosed as having a mental illness, excluding dementias (one-fifth of this sample) have been found to use more services than other participants (Wan and Odell, 1980; Coulton and Frost, 1982; Shapiro and Tate, 1985; Branch et al., 1988; Weissert and Cready, 1989). Therefore, these participants were expected to be more likely to be full-time users of day care services. Participants experiencing dementia, one-quarter of users studied, were expected to attend day care only part time. Again, this expectation was based on findings reported in the literature (Palmer, 1983; Mace and Rabins, 1984). The auspice model was not expected to modify the effects of either mental illness or dementia on frequency of attendance.

Having a history of mental illness was found to increase the probability of full-time attendance, and, also as expected, participants who suffered cognitive impairments such as Alzheimer's and related disorders were less likely to attend day care full time. No significant auspice model differences were found for participants with a history of mental illness. However, suffering from dementias and attending an Auspice Model I center improved the chances that a participant would be full time.

It is possible that the model differences observed for participants with dementias might result from a more advanced level of impairment among

Auspice Model I dementia participants compared to those attending Auspice Model II. However, data were not available to test this severity of illness interpretation.

Diagnoses Two other diagnostic groupings previously found to correlate with nursing home use (Scanlon, 1980) were also included: persons who had had a stroke (19.5 percent of this sample), and persons who currently had or had had cancer (2.2 percent of the sample). The participants in both diagnostic groups were expected to be more likely to attend day care full time. No differences in frequency of attendance among persons who had strokes or cancer were expected between Auspice Model I and Auspice Model II center participants when the analysis controlled for functional dependency.

A history of stroke increased the probability of being a full-time participant; however, among those who had had a stroke, Auspice Model I attendance significantly decreased the likelihood of a participant attending day care full time. Conversely, participants who had cancers were significantly less likely to attend day care; however, participants with this diagnosis had an improved chance of being full time if they attended Auspice Model I rather than Auspice Model II centers. It is important to note that this variable had limited dispersion within the sample, which may weaken confidence in these findings.

These effects of type of center attended may be attributed to differences in the recency of these illness among Auspice Model I compared with Auspice Model II participants. For example, among Auspice Model I participants, more recent strokes may reduce participant stamina thereby limiting attendance, while more current cancers might require more frequent supervision among Auspice Model I participants. As with dementias, data on severity of illness, which could have allowed further analyses of model differences in the effect of diagnoses on frequency of attendance, were not available.

Income Income level should capture the ability of potential users to attend full-time service; thus, relatively high income was expected to have a positive sign. Because income data for participants were not available, county per capita income was used as a proxy. Sample county per capita income averaged $12,624, ranging from $8,780 to $16,878 per year.

Per capita income was found to be negatively related to full-time use, although nonlinear in its association. Residents of higher income counties were less likely to be full-time participants, although the negative influence of higher county per capita income increases at a decreasing rate at the highest income levels.

Private Payment   Private pay charge to participants was expected to be negatively associated with participation frequency, because previous findings show that out-of-pocket payments reduce utilization (Manning et al., 1987). An indicator variable, whether or not participants paid their own charges out of pocket, was expected to be negatively associated with full-time use. The price the participant paid for day care would have been preferable, but these data were not available. Because Auspice Model I centers are relatively more expensive than Auspice Model II centers and collection of fees was less aggressively enforced in Auspice Model II centers, the effect of private payment for services was expected to vary by center type. Specifically, participants in Auspice Model I centers who paid privately were expected to be less likely to attend day care full-time when compared with Auspice Model II participants who paid privately.

Approximately 45 percent of all participants were identified as paying some part of charges for their care out of pocket. Contrary to expectations, private payment for care was associated with an increased probability of full-time attendance. As expected, however, those private-paying participants who used Auspice Model I centers had a reduced chance of being full time. The mixed results of an overall positive influence of private payment and the differential effect across models suggest that private payment may be influenced by both collection policies and price. This potential error in variable demonstrates the importance of these considerations for future research, as well as the difficulty of capturing the data accurately.

Question 3.   How does public reimbursement policy affect full-time use? In particular, does Medicaid, as a payor of adult day care, act as a prudent buyer, rationing full-time use to only the most dependent Medicaid-eligible participants?

Because Medicaid payment on a participant's behalf removes cost sharing, some participants who otherwise could not afford to attend regularly were expected to participate full time. Furthermore, removal of cost sharing would, ceterus paribus, lead to more frequent attendance. (While some states also remove cost sharing for participants funded by Title XX and other state programs, in this sample only Medicaid funding was identified as consistently reducing the individual's cost to zero.) Removal of cost sharing alone therefore might lead to the expectation of a positive sign for Medicaid or an increased probability of full-time attendance.

As a prudent buyer, however, Medicaid is likely to impose utilization controls, probably limiting full-time attendance to those whose conditions make it essential. Under these circumstances, Medicaid would show a negative sign, because most of the 22 percent of participants supported by Medicaid are only minimally dependent (44.9 percent of all Medicaid participants were independent in all activities of daily living, although 38 percent of them had either cognitive limitations or histories of mental illness). On the other hand, if Medicaid is a prudent buyer, the interaction of Medicaid and toileting/eating dependency would be positive.

Because Auspice Model I centers serve a more dependent population, Medicaid was expected to have a less dramatic (negative interaction term) effect on frequency of attendance for participants attending such centers.

As expected, participants who had their care paid for by Medicaid were significantly less likely to attend day care full time than participants funded through other sources, with Medicaid reducing the chances of participants of Auspice Model I being full time.

Also as anticipated, among participants with toileting/eating dependencies, having their care paid for by Medicaid improved the odds that they would attend day care full time relative to similar non-Medicaid participants. Finally, Medicaid participants with functional dependencies and attending an Auspice Model I center had decreased a chance of being full time compared with their counterparts in Auspice Model II centers.

These findings suggest that Medicaid is a prudent buyer with frequency of attendance mediated by patient need.

Question 4.   Does availability of transportation increase the likelihood of full-time use?

Transportation to and from the center has been reported to be critical to day care participation (Weissert, 1975; Palmer, 1983). Transportation to and from the center was expected to increase full-time participation for participants of both auspice model centers.

In this sample 19 percent of all day care participants studied attended centers that offered no transportation; 65 percent attended centers that provided transportation to and from the center only; and 16 percent attended centers that provided comprehensive transportation services, that is, to and from the day care center and to other locations. Centers providing transportation did so daily.

While transportation is recognized as an important enabler of service use, it is unclear whether transportation influences frequency of attendance. The findings for transportation, although in the expected positive direction, were not significant. This nonsignificance suggests that while transportation may be important to whether or not a person uses day care service, it appears to be less important in determining how *much* day care a user will use.

Question 5. How do contextual factors such as county age structure, income, density, and competition from other day care centers affect full-time use?

In considering the effect of competition among day care centers and its influence on frequency of attendance, it is necessary to consider the supply of complementary and substitute services within the county and their impact on use. To control for the supply of other services, two proxy measures for service supply were included in the model: region, and the ratio of nursing homes to elderly resident.

Region: The region variable, Northeast (52 percent of sample), was included in the model to capture regional differences including the relatively richer array of supportive services available to elderly individuals in the Northeast compared to the rest of the country. A richer array of services was assumed to offer substitutes to potential day care full-time use, which was expected to produce a negative sign with no differential effect among models. (It is important to note that few centers in the sample were in the midwest or south-central United States.)

As expected, attending a center located in the Northeast was negatively related to full-time attendance, and no significant model differences were found.

Number of nursing homes per elderly county resident: This variable, the second proxy for service supply, ranged from a low of 0.63 homes to a high of 0.88 homes per thousand elderly county residents, with an average of 0.70 homes per thousand. A log transformation of this variable was necessary because of its positively skewed distribution.

It was expected that the higher the number of nursing homes per elderly county resident, the more likely elderly individuals would be to become nursing home residents, and thus the less likely they would be to seek substitute settings such as day care. In addition, those remaining in the community would likely have lower levels of dependency. A negative effect on full-time attendance was thus expected in areas with high nursing home supply. The type of center attended was not expected to influence the effect of supply of nursing homes on frequency of day care attendance.

The results confirmed our expectations. Participants attending centers located in counties with a relatively high number of nursing homes per elderly person were less likely to be full-time attenders when compared to participants in counties with fewer nursing homes per elderly resident. In counties with more nursing homes per elderly resident, use of an Auspice Model I center reduced the chances of attending day care full time in comparison to users of Auspice Model II centers.

Competition among Day Care Centers Increased competition among day care centers might be expected to lead staff to encourage, or at least allow, participants to attend more frequently because a greater supply of day care services would meet more of demand. Competition in general as well as heavy competition were expected to have similar effects on full-time use in both models.

Most day care centers in this sample faced competition from other centers. Fewer than 7 percent of all participants lived in counties with no competing day care centers, and 5 percent lived in areas with more than twice the average number of centers per elderly county resident. The top quarter of the distribution was 0.089 centers per elderly person in the county. From this distribution, two dichotomous variables were created. These represented any competition and heavy competition; heavy competition indicated 0.089 or more centers per elderly person in the county.

As anticipated, attending a center facing any or heavy competition from other day care providers was positively associated with full-time attendance. An unexpected finding was the differential effect of the amount of competition on frequency of participation depending on type of center attended. Specifically, given the existence of any competition, participants in Auspice Model I centers had reduced odds of full-time use compared to users of Auspice Model II centers facing competition. Conversely, in highly competitive areas, participants in Auspice Model I centers had improved chances of being full-time use compared with users of Auspice Model II centers in highly competitive environments.

This differential influence of competition raises several possible explanations. Explanations consistent with a concept of provider-induced demand include: Auspice Model I programs may assert more influence on frequency of attendance by existing participants when the pool of potential users is limited by more intense competition in highly competitive markets; or Auspice Model II programs may relax their eligibility criteria to include less dependent participants (who attend less frequently) to increase the pool of potential users.

Additional detail on the type of centers that are in competition (e.g., the number of Auspice Model I and number of Auspice Model II centers in a county) may help clarify these issues.

Age Structure of County County age structure was included as a proxy to control for potential demand for services. As noted, participants attending a center that was located in a county with an older age structure were more likely to attend day care full time than day care users in counties with younger age structures. Participants in counties with older age structures had a decreased likelihood of being full time if they used an Auspice Model I center than if they used an Auspice Model II center.

Population Density   County population density was included to capture the potential demand within easy travel distance of centers (proximity of potential demanders to service) in areas of high population per square mile; dense areas were expected to produce more users. But more users do not necessarily equal more full-time users, both because of the richer variety and number of services typically available in highly urbanized areas and because more participants demanding service may lead center staff to discourage full-time use except when absolutely necessary. Therefore, population density was expected to be negatively associated with full-time use (no model differences were anticipated).

Among the sampled counties, population density averaged 552 people per square mile, ranging from a low of 2.7 to a high of 3602. Approximately 61 percent of the participants lived in high-density counties. Based on the skewed distribution of participants on this measure, an indicator variable was constructed for high-density areas ("high density" was defined as being above the median of 102 persons per square mile), and the effect was expected to be negative.

Population density significantly decreased the likelihood of full-time attendance and, as anticipated, no differences were detected between models.

Question 6.   How does percent of capacity used affect use? Do full centers ration full-time use to allow more participants access to services? Because most centers operate below capacity, are patterns likely to change if expanded public subsidies increase demand, allowing more centers to operate closer to capacity?

Center Operating Capacity   Because most centers (85 percent) were operating below their capacity (in the opinion of their directors), an indicator variable was defined for high use of capacity. ("High use" was defined as operating at 90 percent or more of capacity.) As capacity use rises, full-time use should fall if staff discourage full-time use in favor of trying to meet the needs of more people seeking to participate in the center. Participation at centers operating nearer capacity was significantly less likely to be full time as expected, with no significant difference in this effect across center types.

An interaction term was included to capture the multiplicative effect of a center operating at or near its capacity in a high-density area, and was expected to be even more strongly negative than either variable alone. No model differential was expected for either capacity used or the interaction of capacity used with population density.

Results confirmed our hypothesis regarding the multiplicative effects common to both center types, that is, attending a center located in a high-density county where the center is operating at or near capacity was associated with a significantly decreased likelihood of full-time attendance.

Summary of Findings

Variables associated with an increased probability of full-time attendance for day care participants included:

- being age 85 or older
- having a history of nursing home use
- having a history of mental illness
- having a history of stroke
- being dependent in toileting, eating, or both, *and* being subsidized by Medicaid
- being a private payor
- attending a center that was located in a county with older age structure
- attending a center facing competition from other day care providers.

Each of these positive predictors was statistically significant and in the expected direction.

Comparing the two models, participants with the characteristics identified as positive above also had improved chances of attending day care full time if they used a Auspice Model I center rather than as Auspice Model II center, with the following exceptions: being age 85 or older, prior nursing home use, history of stroke, private pay, or competition among day care centers except in heavily competitive counties. Some of these differences may result from differences in the severity of illness or recency of events among Auspice Model I participants; for example, stroke or more recent institutionalization may reduce a participant's stamina. The private pay differential attendance by center may reflect either collection policy differences or the effect of higher costs/charges at Auspice Model I centers. The effects of competition in markets that are not highly competitive is somewhat more perplexing, and suggest that Auspice Model I centers do not respond until competition has reached some critical threshold level.

Characteristics associated with a reduced probability of full-time attendance for the full sample included:

- having impaired mobility
- having Alzheimer's disease or a related dementia
- attending a center located in the Northeast
- attending a center located in a high per capita income county

- attending a center located in a county with a relatively high number of nursing homes per elderly person
- attending a center located in a high-density county, especially if the center is operating at or near capacity.

Comparing the two models, mobility impairments or suffering dementias, characteristics identified as negative above, improved the odds of attending day care full time if the participant used an Auspice Model I center. No significant differences (by center type) in frequency of attendance were found for participants living in the northeast or in high-population density areas, or attending programs operating at or near capacity.

For daycare users living in areas with a high number of nursing homes per capita, use of Auspice Model I centers further decreased the chances of full-time attendance. This model differential is consistent with the expectation that a greater relative supply of nursing homes depletes the potential demand pool of participants with functional dependencies, an effect that would be most obvious among Auspice Model I centers, which serve a higher proportion of these types of individuals.

Conclusions

These data suggest that frequency of day care attendance is influenced by auspice model, participant characteristics, and community variables. Transportation, the single center service introduced in the model, does not appear to influence frequency of participation, although access to transportation was previously found to have a substantial impact on use or nonuse of day care services.

Medicaid, as a subsidizer of day care, does appear to be a prudent buyer, with frequency of participation sensitive to participant needs.

In addition, center characteristics such as competition among day care providers and the efficiency of service delivery (capacity of maximal operations achieved) do appear to influence frequency of participation. To fully understand these contextual and market effects, research that tests causal relationships, using more direct measures of price and more detailed data on service supply and competition, should be employed.

These results do suggest, however, that factors influencing frequency of adult day care participation are in most respects similar to those important in understanding use of other health care services by the elderly. Most findings were consistent with other researchers' findings for other types of services, and in general were in the expected direction.

One finding unique to this study, however, was that auspices of the center being attended may alter the effect of a participant's characteristics on frequency of attendance. For example, although stroke participants were more likely than nonstroke participants to attend full time, this was less often the case if they attended a Model I rather than a Model II center. In most instances, those attending centers affiliated with nursing homes and rehabilitation hospitals (Model I) attended day care less frequently than participants of centers affiliated with other types of agencies (Model II).

THREE

PARTICIPANT AND CAREGIVER SATISFACTION WITH ADULT DAY CARE

ADULT DAY CARE is distinctive within the range of health care options available to the elderly because it is community based. This distinctiveness raises interesting questions in identifying the qualities that attract participants to day care centers, as well as the qualities that determine the satisfaction of participants and caregivers with the centers. Ultimately, the success of day care rests on factors that predict satisfaction and contribute to continued utilization. In a consumer approach to medical care, satisfaction with the service can be conceptualized as an intervening variable between need for care and continued utilization and cooperation with the medical care provider.

This chapter reports and discusses the findings of the national survey that concern factors contributing to satisfaction with adult day care. The measures and analyses of satisfaction reflect participants' and caregivers' reported perceptions about their experiences with their center, not an objective rating of the services rendered. As Ware et al. (1983) has pointed out, satisfaction ratings are subjective and represent the affective component in the decision to use a given health care. This affective rating was expected to be related to participants' personal characteristics as well as to the structural conditions that make it easy or difficult to take advantage of the services.

Review of the Literature

Little attention has been focused on the factors associated with satisfaction with adult day care centers per se, but patient satisfaction with health care in general has received a great deal of attention in recent years. In this context, satisfaction is defined as satisfaction with the care received, not with improvement in general life satisfaction or contentment with life in general.

The literature on patient satisfaction yields no consistent profile of the satisfied client. Weiss (1988) reported that the inconsistency may result from the variety of samples studied and methods used to measure satisfaction. Also contributing to this inconsistency is the variety of health care modes evaluated. Often a particular form of primary care is evaluated, or types of primary health care plans are compared, or physicians' services in general are considered.

Demographic factors have most frequently been used as predictive variables in studies of satisfaction. These variables include subjective health ratings, source of payment, and, in the case of health maintenance organizations, continuity in the health care received. In general, these variables parallel Andersen and Aday's categories of predisposing, enabling, and need designed to be used in health care utilization (Aday & Andersen, 1974).

The demographic factors that function as predisposing variables include age, race, marital status, and gender. Several studies found older patients to be more satisfied (Pope, 1978; Ware et al., 1978; Gray, 1980; DiMatteo & Hays, 1980; Linn et al., 1982; Zastowny et al., 1983), while other studies found age to be nonsignificant (Weiss, 1988) or inversely related to satisfaction (Hulka et al., 1975). Some studies found white people to be more satisfied than black people with physicians' care (Gray, 1980; Hulka et al., 1975; Linn et al., 1982), and Zastowny et al. (1983) reported opposite results; however, others have found no relationship between race and satisfaction (Weiss, 1988; Greenley & Schoenherr, 1981; Marquis et al., 1983).

Studies that found a relationship between gender and satisfaction usually reported that women had higher levels of satisfaction than men (Ware et al., 1978; DiMatteo & Hays, 1980; Zastowny et al., 1983). The relationship of marital status to satisfaction has been less frequently analyzed, but Tessler and Mechanic (1975) found married persons to be less satisfied with medical care than unmarried persons.

Several researchers have looked at other personal attitudes as predisposing the individual toward satisfaction, including the level of life satisfaction the person expresses. It is argued that some people have a negative view of life in general, and their attitude toward medical care is just one aspect of the total picture.

While the utilization literature shows the importance of need as a predictor of use, the picture is not as clear when the dependent variable is patient satisfaction. Even in terms of health status and its relationship to satisfaction with care, the findings are diverse. Romm and Hulka (1979) and DiMatteo and Hays (1980) found no relationship, while Tessler and Mechanic (1975) and Pope (1978) found that persons in good health generally felt more satisfied with the care they received.

While individuals' characteristics have been found to be important (Zastowny et al., 1983), several studies have placed greater emphasis on the organizational characteristics of the health care providers or on factors that enable a person to use the service. Much of the research on client satisfaction compares primary care clinics, where access to a regular physician is a major issue, to care under a single physician. Other studies have focused on the type of payment plan. For instance, Tessler and Mechanic (1975) found that enrollees in fee-for-service insurance plans were more satisfied than enrollees in prepaid group practice plans.

Other than the findings just discussed, research on satisfaction with health care in general has little applicability to adult day care. Elderly people in search of day care may have specific needs that prompt their use of the service, and those persons with certain types of health problems may be greater users and more or less satisfied customers as a result of their specific health limitations. There is no general, theory connected with previous studies that can be applied to the day care setting.

Day care, however, is interesting because various levels of societal organization merge therein; that is, individuals, family units, community organizations, and health care institutions become interrelated. Certainly individual characteristics are important: age, race, sex, marital status, living arrangements, etc. Types of payment, private or Medicaid, are also important, as well as other enabling characteristics, such as transportation to the center. But there are also questions of auspices or type of day care, whether the center is primarily rehabilitation oriented or oriented more toward social service. While hospitals and all physicians are licensed, all day care centers are not. Does the oversight of a regulatory agency that is necessary for licensure lead to greater participant satisfaction? Does the size of the day care center (both in terms of size of staff and number of participants) make a difference to the participant? Is the number of services a matter of concern?

Finally, day care occupies a position between completely independent living and institutionalized living. Does the market supply of nursing home beds affect the utilization of day care, and if it does, is this a positive influence on participants or a negative one in terms of their satisfaction with the service? Does the supply of adult day care centers or the existence of a waiting list lead to competition for clients or a laissez-faire attitude toward the satisfaction of the participants? Thus, an evaluation of adult day care necessitates focusing more on the community and selecting a broader range of variables than studies of other types of patient satisfaction.

Measurement Issues

Several major attempts to refine the measurement of satisfaction have been made, particularly in the work of Hulka et al. and of Ware et al. (see Zastowny et al., 1983, for an overview). Measurement of satisfaction has ranged from a single item assessing overall satisfaction to a number of items that are then factor analyzed and summed into scales. The latter approach emphasizes the various domains of satisfaction. For example, the work of Hulka and colleagues discusses three conceptual dimensions: the personal qualities of physicians; the professional qualities and competence of physicians; and the cost and convenience of services. Ware and his colleagues, using factor-analytical techniques, found 18 dimensions to satisfaction but highlighted only 4 of these: access to care, continuity of care, availability of services, and physician conduct.

Although a considerable amount of work has focused on the measurement of satisfaction, the relative importance of each of the established domains or whether one type of satisfaction is more relevant to a particular type of medical care compared to another type have not been ascertained. Because research on adult day care is fairly new, our study examined the components that make day care unique. Adult day care centers, as distinct from primary care clinics, offer a center and a variety of staff personnel that work with the participant. Because adult day care is community based and the population is elderly, transportation to and from the center can be extremely important. Other factors, such as center hours, quality of food, and quality of physical surroundings, may all affect the elderly person's satisfaction with day care. Lawton and Nahemow (1979) have argued that older persons are more influenced by the environment than younger persons, and to the extent that this is true, one would expect the environment of the day care center to be important in determining satisfaction with care.

Data and Measures

Data on participant satisfaction were derived from the subsample of participant interviews. Participants were asked the following questions concerning aspects of adult day care:

1. I'd like to know how you feel about the overall center here; Would you say that you are satisfied, partly satisfied or dissatisfied? (1 = satisfied; 0 = partly satisfied or dissatisfied).
2. Now think about the amount of individual attention that you get here;

Would you say that you are satisfied, partly satisfied, or dissatisfied? (1 = satisfied; 0 = partly satisfied or dissatisfied).

3. How often can you count on the staff to do what they are supposed to do for you? Would you say that you can count on the staff most of the time, some of the time, or can't you count on them at all? (1 = most or all of the time; 0 = some of the time or can't count on them at all).

4. Would you say that you are satisfied, partly satisfied, or not satisfied with the transportation system that brings you here and takes you home? (1 = satisfied; 0 = partly satisfied or dissatisfied).

5. Would you say the center's hours are too long, too short, or about right? (1 = about right; 0 = too long or too short).

6. How about the food here; Would you say that you are satisfied, partly satisfied, or dissatisfied with the food here? (1 = satisfied; 0 = partly satisfied or dissatisfied).

7. Is it too hot or too cold for you here? Would you say that it is often, sometimes, or never too hot or too cold? (1 = never; 0 = often or sometimes).

8. Does this place seem crowded to you? Would you say this place often, sometimes, or rarely seems crowded? (1 = rarely; 0 = sometimes or often);

9. Do you think it is too noisy here? Would you say that it is often, sometimes, or rarely ever too noisy here? (1 = rarely or never; 0 = sometimes or often).

For the two Auspice Model categories, these items were then factor analyzed, and all but one were selected as an indicator of one of three components of participant satisfaction. The analysis excludes participants of Special-Purpose Centers because of their small sample size. These factors were later used in a multivariate analysis.

The demographic variables included age of the respondent measured in chronological years, living arrangements (1 = alone), marital status (1 = married), race (1 = white), and gender (1 = male).

One measure of participant attitudes is included in the analysis. This is a global measure of life satisfaction: In general, how satisfying do you find the way you are spending your life these days? Would you call it completely satisfying, pretty satisfying, or not very satisfying? (1 = completely satisfying; 0 = pretty satisfying or not very satisfying).

In addition the Short Portable Mental Status Questionnaire (Pfeiffer, 1975) was used to assess mental status and used as a control measure in the multivariate analysis. The 10-question instrument includes such items as identifying the current date and day of the week, identifying the current president of the United States, and recalling the mother's maiden name.

The need for adult day care was assessed by the level of dependency the older person was experiencing in the tasks of daily living. Items assessing dependency in bathing, dressing, mobility, toileting, and eating were summed and scored.

Two variables generally associated with enabling factors were also included in the analysis. Both are dummy variables for type of payment, asking whether payment was entirely by Medicaid or entirely by private payment (1 = Medicaid only, and 1 = private pay only).

Seven variables unique to day care were used. These variables do not easily fall under the headings of predisposing, enabling, and need, but focus instead on the center's service orientation and its role in providing a custodial form of care that intervenes between the home and an institution. First, a dummy variable representing the Auspice Model of the center was included in the analysis. The variable was coded so that 1 = Auspice Model I and 0 = Model II.

The remaining variables included the number of unoccupied nursing home beds in the county per thousand persons over 65; a dummy variable for whether the center was licensed or not (1 = licensed); a summed score for the number of therapeutic services offered by the center; the presence of therapeutic staff in terms of a nurse and a therapist (2 = both, 1 = one or the other, 0 = none); the total number of additional staff members; and a computation of the average number of participants attending the site per day. Both the number of participants and the number of staff were used as independent variables. An alternative would be to construct a ratio of staff to participants. However, the advantage of separate independent variables is that we can identify whether it is the number of participants or the number of staff that makes a difference when all other things are equal.

The number of available nursing home beds indicates the market in which the day care center is competing. Because we are controlling for need, this variable, if significant, reflects how the supply of beds influences institutional versus community-based care. When no beds are available, people who are more dependent in their health care needs might be forced into day care while they wait for institutional placement. At the same time, a superfluous number of beds might also indicate where the community has placed economic resources. Licensing indicates that the center has met the requirements of the state or county and that day care is developed sufficiently in the area for regulatory standards to be established.

The availability of services should attract participants to the center while increasing expectations and demand for their delivery. The number of staff, apart from a registered nurse or therapist, should also be related to participants' satisfaction, as more staff, controlling for number of attendees, should make it possible for the elderly participant to receive more personal attention. Finally, the size of the day care center as indicated by the average number of persons who attend per day may increase demands on personnel and lower the attention each participant receives.

Participant Satisfaction with Adult Day Care

DESCRIPTIVE FINDINGS

The participants in this analysis ranged in age from 65 to 96 years with a mean age of 79. Approximately 34 percent lived alone; 29 percent were married, and 76 percent were white. The range on the activities of daily living (ADL) dependency index was from 0 to 4; the mean was less than 1, indicating that this group of elderly people was generally capable of performing ADLs independently. The Mental Status measure ranged from 0 to 10, with a mean of 6.06. Forty-three percent of the participants were paying for day care entirely by private funds, while another 11.5 percent were entirely covered by Medicaid. Twenty-one percent of the participants were attending a day care center that can be characterized as post acute, and close to 57 percent were in a licensed center. Most participants in the sample were satisfied with life (mean = 2.25 where 3 = satisfied), and 60 percent reported a postive change in their lives as a result of attending day care.

As in most studies of health care, participants were found to be highly satisfied. Participant satisfaction with the overall center ran particularly high; 91 percent reported that they were satisfied and 92 percent said that they were satisfied with the attention of the staff. Similar percentages of participants reported satisfaction with center hours and transportation to and from the center. There was greater variation when the participants were asked to evaluate the quality of food and the noisiness, crowdedness, or temperature of the center. Approximately three-fourths reported being satisfied with the food; slightly fewer than three-fourths were satisfied with the temperature and three-fifths with the noise level. The lowest level of satisfaction was reported regarding the crowdedness of centers; even so, slightly more than half were very satisfied. Slightly less than one-fourth of the sample were completely satisfied with all aspects of day care. Summary statistics are presented in Table 3.1.

MULTIVARIATE ANALYSIS

Satisfaction with day care was assessed by nine items, which were then factor analyzed to determine the dimensions of satisfaction. The factor analysis identified three major factors. One factor reflected the structural dimension of day care and was most highly associated with the center

Table 3.1
Percentage of Participants Satisfied with Aspects of Adult Day Care

Aspect	Percent
Satisfied with overall program	91.0
Can rely on staff	92.5
Satisfied with amount of individual attention	91.8
Believe useful things are done at center	75.5
Satisfied with transportation	94.2
Satisfied with center food	76.4
Satisfied with lack of crowding	53.5
Satisfied with noise level	60.4
Satisfied with program hours	90.8
Satisfied with temperature in center	71.8
Totally satisfied with all items	23.8

hours, transportation to and from the center, the quality of the food, and whether the center temperature was satisfactory. A second factor focused on satisfaction with the center itself and with its personnel. A third factor, which appears to be a measure of center milieu, was indicated by the items dealing with crowdedness and noisiness, and this was interpreted as favoring a calm environment and a low level of turmoil.

The four items reflecting satisfaction with center structure had an overall reliability as measured by Cronbach's alpha of .55, the two-item scale measuring more intrinsic satisfaction with the center and staff had a reliability of .58, and the third index had a reliability of .73. These three components of satisfaction explained 51.6 percent of the variation in the nine items, and they constitute the dependent variables in the analyses described below.

BIVARIATE ASSOCIATIONS

Examination of satisfaction with the structural characteristics of the center (hours, food, transportation, and center temperature) showed older, white, male, and married participants to be more satisfied with the center than the young-old, nonwhite, female, and single participants. Those who lived alone were least satisfied.

The participants who had previous nursing home experience in a skilled facility also reported higher levels of satisfaction with day care than participants who had never been institutionalized. It appears that those who have been institutionalized appreciate care that permits them to continue living somewhat independently.

Participants who have endocrine, nutritonal, or metabolic disorders, excluding diabetes, tend to be most satisfied with the structural conditions of the center, including the quality of the food and the center hours. Participants who appear to be less satisfied are those who experience hypertension or poorly defined symptoms, and those suffering from cancer. The latter two types of participants appear to have special problems that are not addressed as well in the adult day care center as are other types of problems, or perhaps are less satisfied in general because of their medical conditions.

Participants who privately paid their total day care expenses were more satisfied than those who received a subsidy, and participants whose day care expenses were paid for entirely by Medicaid were the least satisfied. The more participants can pay their own way, the more satisfied they are with the structural conditions of the day care center. This finding probably reflects both the objective conditions of the center and the quality of what can be purchased and the likelihood that dissatisfied private payors have "voted with their feet" and left the center.

In terms of psychological measures, participants who scored lower on the short portable mental status questionnaire expressed lower levels of satisfaction. However, the zero-order relationship between life satisfaction in general and satisfaction with day care was negative. This latter finding was unexpected, because the argument usually advanced is that people who are happier with life in general would be positively predisposed in their evaluation of specific services. Our finding would argue that such people are better able to be critical of a specific condition.

Two center-level variables were associated with participant satisfaction: whether the center had a participant waiting list, and the size of the center's staff. The centers with the largest staff, over and above a nurse and therapist, had more satisfied participants, while centers with waiting lists had less satisfied members. It may be that day care centers with waiting lists do not need to worry about losing their customers. The supply of potential participants is large enough that the center need not upgrade to be fully utilized. However, competition does have some effect, for participants in communities with many adult day care centers were found to be more satisfied. Competition for clients encourages centers to make hours and transportation convenient for the elderly and complements the finding that centers with waiting lists had less satisfied clients. In addition, multiple day care centers may indicate communities that are more organized to provide adult day care, raising the level of satisfaction of the elderly participants. The results are summarized in Table 3.2.

Table 3.2
Variables Related to Structural Satisfaction with Program

	Correlation	Significance
Individual-Level Variables		
Age	.372	.000
White	.516	.000
Male	.152	.057
Married	.307	.001
Previously admitted to skilled nursing facility	.343	.000
ADL dependency	.050	.302
Lives alone	−.340	.000
Life satisfaction	−.207	.016
Stroke	.034	.363
Circulatory system disorders (excluding hypertension and stroke)	.010	.458
Respiratory system disorders	−.026	.395
Hypertension	−.208	.015
Cancer	−.162	.047
Symptoms (poorly defined condition)	−.224	.010
Endocrine, nutritional metabolic disorders (excluding diabetes)	.280	.002
Private pay only	.396	.000
Medicaid only	−.170	.047
Mental health status	−.224	.012
Center-Level Variables		
Auspice Model I	.018	.426
Therapeutic services	.043	.342
Presence of a therapeutic staff	.077	.217
Size of staff	.350	.000
Center is licensed	.119	.130
Center receives Medicaid funds	.070	.239
Center has waiting list	−.455	.000
Average daily attendance	−.046	.323
Community-Level Variables		
Number of unoccupied nursing home beds	−.135	.081
Number of other adult day care centers	.223	.010

Some of the variables related to satisfaction with the structure of the center show a similar relationship with intrinsic satisfaction with the center. Older, married, male participants have higher levels of both types of satisfaction than younger, single, female participants. In addition, day care participants who have been in skilled nursing homes also report high levels of satisfaction with the center. Other participant-level variables that relate similarly to the two kinds of satisfaction include clients with poorly defined symptoms who are less satisfied, and clients with endocrine, nutritional, or metabolic disorders who are more likely to be satisfied than others. Other similarities include, at the center level, the size of staff, and at the community level, the number of adult day care centers. Both are positively associated with satisfaction.

Two variables are significantly related to the two types of satisfaction but in opposite directions. Concern about a general Pollyanna effect (i.e., that those whose views on life are generally positive will evaluate centers more highly) receives support when internal satisfaction with the center is measured. Because of the positive correlation between the two attitudes, one should control for a measure of general life satisfaction in multivariate analysis of intrinsic satisfaction. The other variable with an opposite effect is that of race; nonwhites reported higher levels of satisfaction with the center itself than reported by whites. It may be that centers serving minority persons, although possibly not as convenient in terms of hours and transportation or quality of food, enrich the lives of minority persons to a greater extent than centers that serve majority members. At the same time, five variables associated with intrinsic satisfaction were not related to structural satisfaction: (1) functional dependence, (2) having had a stroke, (3) circulatory problems, (4) presence of therapeutic services, and (5) whether the center was licensed or not.

It is interesting to look at this set of zero-order correlations. With the exception of stroke patients, participants who need help and who could benefit from rehabilitative assistance appear to find adult day care particularly satisfying, with licensed centers and those offering the greater number of services having more satisfied participants. These latter centers appear able to satisfy a broad range of clients. The results are summarized in Table 3.3.

The third factor, satisfaction with the general milieu of the center, shows some very different patterns. Men, married participants, and participants who had been in skilled nursing facilities were less satisfied with the calmness of the environment and seemed to perceive more turmoil. These three variables (gender, marital status, and having been in a skilled facility) are interrelated. The men are probably able to leave the nursing home because they have wives to serve as primary caregivers, but the wives need assistance from the day care center. It may be that the change to day

Table 3.3
Variables Related to Intrinsic Satisfaction with Program

	Correlation	Significance
Individual-Level Variables		
Age	.107	.000
White	−.155	.047
Male	.195	.016
Married	.137	.066
Previously admitted to skilled nursing facility	.210	.015
ADL dependency	.128	.082
Lives alone	.090	.163
Life satisfaction	.236	.005
Stroke	−.123	.090
Circulatory system disorders (excluding hypertension and stroke)	.123	.090
Respiratory system disorders	.102	.134
Hypertension	−.074	.212
Cancer	.058	.265
Symptoms (poorly defined condition)	−.372	.000
Endocrine, nutritional metabolic disorders (excluding diabetes)	.125	.087
Private pay only	.053	.296
Medicaid only	.116	.119
Mental health status	−.103	.137
Center-Level Variables		
Auspice Model I	−.041	.327
Therapeutic services	.206	.019
Presence of therapeutic staff	−.030	.373
Size of staff	.228	.007
Center is licensed	.265	.004
Center receives Medicaid funds	.070	.229
Center has waiting list	.153	.065
Average daily attendance	.112	.119
Community-Level Variables		
Number of unoccupied nursing home beds	−.059	.261
Number of adult day care centers	.155	.044

care creates more of a disturbance in their lives. At the same time, those who are currently more dependent are in centers where they are satisfied with the overall milieu. Participants with circulatory problems, as well as those with better mental health, were satisfied with the overall milieu; however, participants who have endocrine, nutritional, or metabolic problems were less satisfied.

When terms of payment was related to satisfaction with the milieu of the day care, privately paying participants apparently expected more and were dissatisfied, whereas Medicaid-only participants were generally satisfied.

Center-level variables were correlated, as expected, with a calm environment. Auspice Model I centers were more often satisfying in terms of quietude than the Auspice Model II centers. Licensed centers, which are also those that receive Medicaid funds, were less satisfying in terms of noise and crowdedness. Centers with large staffs and a high average number of attendees were also less satisfying. Somewhat surprisingly, the zero-order correlation between the number of adult day care centers and satisfaction with the milieu was negative. The more centers, the greater the activity at the centers. It may be that communities with a large number of adult day care centers are particularly active in terms of services and activities that take place in adult day care. These results are summarized in Table 3.4.

REGRESSION ANALYSIS

Many of the variables are highly intercorrelated (such as marital status, living alone, gender, having been in a skilled nursing home, and size of staff). Married men were more likely to have been in a skilled nursing home, and those who had been in a nursing home were likely to be in a day care center with a large staff. It is probable that marital status was a crucial factor in the men being able to leave the skilled facility and return to community living, albeit with support. The spouse provided enough care that the husband could leave the institutionalized setting, yet she was unable to take complete care of him. Day care participants who had been in a skilled facility were more numerous in communities having more centers. Thus the variables included in the regression analysis had to be a very small subset of those variables previously discussed.

The three types of satisfaction also measured different aspects of day care, and it is not surprising that the prediction equation for each should therefore vary as well. The analysis was conducted on the cases for which there was valid information on all variables, which ranged from 105 to 116 of the 132 cases available for analysis. Missing data occurred primarily when one of the attitude questions was not answered.

Table 3.4
Variables Related to Satisfaction with Calmness of the Environment

	Correlation	Significance
Individual-Level Variables		
Age	.120	.092
White	.021	.410
Male	−.316	.000
Married	−.436	.000
Previously admitted to skilled nursing facility	−.572	.000
ADL dependency	.332	.000
Lives alone	.122	.088
Life satisfaction	.110	.115
Stroke	.105	.122
Circulatory system disorders (excluding hypertension and stroke)	.365	.000
Respiratory system disorders	.061	.252
Hypertension	.008	.466
Cancer	−.002	.492
Symptoms (poorly defined condition)	.000	.499
Endocrine, nutritional metabolic disorders (excluding diabetes)	−.527	.000
Private pay only	−.302	.001
Medicaid only	.192	.022
Mental health status	.169	.034
Center-Level Variables		
Auspice Model I	.238	.004
Therapeutic services	−.198	.022
Presence of therapeutic staff	.008	.464
Size of staff	−.590	.000
Center is licensed	−.300	.001
Center receives Medicaid funds	−.284	.002
Center has waiting list	.133	.092
Average daily attendance	−.278	.001
Community-Level Variables		
Number of unoccupied nursing home beds	−.064	.237
Number of adult day care centers	−.427	.000

First, all the variables selected for the equations come from the domains of individual characteristics, center characteristics, and community characteristics. However, the specific variables from each of these domains that predict satisfaction after controlling for other variables from the other two domains are often different. Predictors of structural satisfaction were race (white), age, living alone, and having symptoms associated with a poorly defined condition. These four variables predicted 37 percent of the variation in satisfaction with the structural conditions of the center. Those who lived alone or who had illness symptoms were less satisfied with the structural conditions of day care and appeared to be more sensitive to such issues as transportation, center hours, quality of food, and center temperature. Whites and older participants proved to be the most satisfied with the structural conditions of the center.

These findings seem logical. Elderly participants who live alone may be particularly handicapped in finding a way to the center, and the convenience of center hours may be paramount to their getting there. For participants with aches and pains, the inconvenience of either the schedule or transportation could add just enough difficulty to the situation to make them decide that getting to the center would be just too difficult; similarly, a temperature comfortable for these less healthy participants might not be comfortable for others. These results are summarized in Table 3.5.

To measure satisfaction with the intrinsic quality of the center, it was necessary to conduct a logit analysis because the split on this variable was skewed, with 89 percent very satisfied. The equation included the respondent's general life satisfaction, the size of the staff over and above one nurse and one therapist, and whether the participant had illness symptoms. These variables were particularly effective in predicting intrinsic satisfaction; however, most participants were satisfied with the center and the staff. Thus, this aspect of satisfaction had the least amount of overall variation.

Table 3.5
Regression Coefficients for Satisfaction with Structural Conditions

	Coefficient	Standardized coefficient	p value
Lives alone	−.491	−.255	.002
White	.741	.338	.000
Symptoms poorly defined condition	−.758	−.188	.018
Age	.033	.235	.010
Adjusted R^2 = .37 (n = 105)			

Participants who have illness symptoms but no well-defined health problem appear to be the most difficult to satisfy intrinsically as well as structurally. They do not feel well, yet there is no clear diagnosis. Their health complaints cannot be classified into an ICD-9 category such as infectious diseases, neoplasms, mental disorders, nervous or other systems, etc., but instead fall into the ICD-9 classification of "symptoms, signs and ill-defined conditions." This includes general symptoms as well as symptoms involving the head and neck, nervous and musculoskeletal systems, cardiovascular system, etc. Such persons responded more negatively to the centers than other types of participants. The number of staff members, over and above one therapist and nurse, did contribute to participant's level of satisfaction. The larger the staff, the more satisfied were the participants with the attention they received and with the center itself. At the same time, the number of attendees had no effect on intrinsic satisfaction, and so this variable was dropped from the analysis.

The effects of symptoms and of the number of staff members on intrinsic satisfaction with the center were independent of the participant's general life satisfaction. These relationships with center satisfaction cannot be attributed to a general "Pollyanna" feeling as they are independent of the relationship between general life satisfaction and program satisfaction. This is not to say that the two types of satisfaction are not correlated—they are. Those persons with positive attitudes toward life in general tended to be more satisfied with their day care center. (The reverse may also be argued; those who are satisfied with the center are also more satisfied with life in general.) There may be a similar but reverse phenomenon going on with those who report symptoms and are less satisfied: Those who are discontented with their health are discontented with the centers. The results are summarized in Table 3.6.

The final component of satisfaction, that of being satisfied with the center's milieu, was analyzed using ordinary least squares, as this variable was normally distributed. Explanatory variables included staff size, average number of attendees, participant age, participant with nervous or endo-

Table 3.6
Coefficients for Intrinsic Satisfaction with Program (Logit Analysis; $n = 115$)

	Coefficient	p value
Life satisfaction	3.381	.001
Size of staff	.733	.001
Symptoms, poorly defined conditions	-6.262	.000

crine system disorders, and whether the participant was privately paying his or her total expenses.

Fifty-four percent of the variation in this measure was explained. The participants were likely to be less satisfied with the noise level and crowdedness when they had endocrine disorders and in instances where there were more staff. In fact, this latter variable had a zero-order correlation of $-.59$ with this dimension of satisfaction. The effect of average daily attendance was also significantly related to dissatisfaction with the center's milieu. This finding illustrates an interesting dilemma for day care centers and directors; a larger staff increases participants' intrinsic satisfaction, for they like the attention they can receive for their needs, but they do not like the accompanying noise and the more crowded feeling.

Compared to subsidized participants, privately paying participants also were less satisfied with the level of noise and crowdedness in day care centers, while older participants and those with nervous system disorders were more satisfied. The results are summarized in Table 3.7.

Satisfaction of Caregivers
with Adult Day Care Centers

Little has been said about caregivers' satisfaction with adult day care. Like participants, however, caregivers were found to be highly satisfied with the centers. Eighty-nine percent of the 110 caregivers in our study reported the highest level of satisfaction measured by a single item giving an overall assessment of the center.

Table 3.7
Regression Coefficients for Satisfaction with Calmness of the Environment

	Coefficient	Standardized coefficient	p value
Age	.047	.339	.000
Size of staff	$-.019$	$-.238$	.069
Average number of attendees	$-.024$	$-.201$	.020
Private paying only	$-.382$	$-.208$	.019
Nervous system disorders	.340	.156	.031
Endocrine, nutritional, metabolic problems (excluding diabetes)	$-.653$	$-.327$	.008
Adjusted $R^2 = .54$ ($n = 103$)			

Many associations were investigated to find predictors of caregiver satisfaction. These associations included the relationship of the participant to the caregiver, the number of hours of caregiving the person provided, the time caregivers had available for themselves, whether the caregiver worked, and the type of help caregivers provided for the participant.

Very few of these variables showed any relationship with the caregiver's satisfaction. Sons and daughters appeared to be slightly less satisfied with day care than spouses, siblings, or other categories of caregivers. Caregivers were less satisfied with day care if they used the time the participant was in day care to clean their own homes, but the more important caregiver variable was whether the caregivers themselves worked. Working was assessed as 1 for part-time workers, 2 for full-time, and 0 for otherwise. The more hours the caregiver worked, the more satisfied he or she was with day care services. If caregivers reported not having had enough time for themselves before the family member was in day care, they tended to be more satisfied with the overall center. The number of hours of help the caregiver provided, however, showed no clearly consistent pattern.

Some participant characteristics affected the caregiver's feelings. Caregivers of participants who were older, were married, suffered from stroke, circulatory problems, cancer, or illness symptoms, and were privately paying all reported less satisfaction. Caregivers were more critical of licensed centers, of centers in communities where there were greater numbers of day care centers, and of centers having numerous staff and services. Only in the case of more dependent participants were the cargivers more satisfied.

These zero-order correlations, presented in Table 3.8, are a bit surprising and must be interpreted cautiously because no special circumstances are taken into account. The satisfaction variable is highly skewed, and by far most caregivers were found to be completely satisfied. It may well be that the more that is offered by the day care center, the more there is on which it can be evaluated.

The multivariate analysis was conducted on the 96 cases for which there were complete data. Logit analysis was used because of the highly skewed nature of the dependent variable. The analysis showed an interesting effect, a relationship between type of center, mode of payment, a working caregiver, and satisfaction of the caregiver (Table 3.9). If the participant attended an Auspice Model I center, centers in which participants tended to be most functionally dependent, caregivers were more satisfied. Caregivers were also more satisfied if they themselves worked, whether full time or part time, with full-time workers being most satisfied. More critical caregivers were those of privately paying participants. The analysis was extended to examine whether caregivers of participants with different illnesses were equally satisfied. These results are presented in Table 3.10.

Table 3.8
Variables Related to Satisfaction of Caregivers

	Correlation	Significance
Individual-Level Variables		
Caregiver is an offspring	−.125	.096
Caregiver works	.199	.019
Caregiver uses time for cleaning	−.165	.043
Caregivers did *not* have time for themselves before day care	.148	.095
Age of participant	−.184	.025
Participant is married	−.155	.053
Participant has had a stroke	−.133	.083
Participant has circulatory problems (excluding hypertension and stroke)	−.250	.004
Cancer	−.546	.000
Symptoms (poorly defined condition)	−.134	.082
Endocrine, nutritional metabolic disorders (excluding diabetes)	.008	.468
Participant is dependent in ADL	.130	.095
Participant is private pay only	−.239	.009
Center-Level Variables		
Auspice Model I	.082	.199
Therapeutic services	−.136	.100
Size of staff	−.256	.003
Center is licensed	−.185	.041
Community-Level Variables		
Number of other adult day care centers	−.204	.016

Caregivers of participants who have cancer or illness symptoms face an added burden and are less satisfied. Caregivers of cancer patients may be struggling with ever-increasing dependency while caregivers of elderly with poorly defined conditions must also cope with the dissatisfaction of the participant.

Conclusions

These evaluations of center participants' and caregivers' perceptions of adult day care centers show high levels of satisfaction; adult day care has

Table 3.9
Coefficients for Satisfaction of Caregivers (Logit Analysis; n = 96)

	Coefficient	p value
Auspice Model I	2.021	.022
Caregiver works	1.191	.018
Participant is private paying	− 2.274	.004

been well received. Adult day care appears to be meeting the needs of its clientele, particularly caregivers who are trying to balance family commitments with their own jobs. Contemporary society has seen major changes in the roles of women and their increased involvement in the labor force. As a result, although women remain the primary caregivers, fewer women are available for full-time caregiving. Day care appears to be contributing to the resolution of this dilemma, and one can expect the industry to grow.

Although most participants were highly satisfied, specific variables unique to people's lives lead them to discriminate among various aspects of the day care center. For example, participants who are satisfied with the intrinsic quality of the center, as is true, for example, of the participants attending centers with large staffs, may appear less satisfied with the calmness of the environment. Taken together, these findings lead one to believe that satisfaction with one aspect counterbalances dissatisfaction with another; thus, participants continued to attend and remained satisfied overall.

Of the three measures, the center milieu (its noisiness and crowdedness) appeared to be most problematic for elderly participants. Although these factors probably can be improved, solutions may involve trade-offs with efforts to reduce costs by operating with a larger daily census.

Participants with symptoms, signs, or poorly defined conditions appear

Table 3.10
Coefficients for Satisfaction of Caregivers Controlling for Participants' Medical Problems
(Logit Analysis; n = 96)

	Coefficient	p value
Auspice Model I	1.731	.101
Caregiver works	.788	.133
Participant private paying	− 1.360	.133
Symptoms, poorly defined conditions	− 1.829	.033
Cancer	− 3.564	.008

to be the most consistently less satisfied, as are their caregivers. These persons should not be arbitrarily dismissed as complainers. The ambiguity of their conditions may mean they are not receiving as much service or that the staff may not know how to help, and decreased attention to their needs could aggravate an already difficult situation. Adult day care personnel should be alert to such situations to determine the most appropriate response to their clients' needs.

FOUR

LICENSURE
AND CERTIFICATION OF
ADULT DAY CARE

IN THIS CHAPTER we examine the extent, scope, and apparent effects of licensure and certification in the adult day care industry, as well as provider attitudes toward regulation.

Requirements for licensure and certification regulate a substantial proportion of adult day care centers. State and local governments establish licensing requirements to ensure that an adult day care center has met minimum standards expected of centers used by the public, and certification serves to align a center's operations with a funding agency's guidelines. State laws generally address standards for licensure, while state and federal grant regulations and statutes (such as the state/federal Medicaid program, the Older Americans Act, and the Social Services Block Grants) set certification standards.

Even though licensure and certification requirements are formulated by different bodies and serve slightly different purposes, they converge at many points. It is common for certifying agencies to require that a center be licensed before certification is granted. Similar requirements for both certification and licensure affect center services, participant eligibility for services, staff composition and numbers, facility characteristics, and hours of operation.

In addition, federal, state, and local laws barring discrimination against the handicapped require actions to eliminate barriers that might restrict access. Section 504 of the Vocational Rehabilitation Act of 1973* is prominent among such statutes. The standards of the American National Standards Institute (ANSI) for barrier-free access are often included in licensure and certification requirements.

*Rehabilitation Act of 1973, Public Law No. 93-112, Sec. 504, 87 Stat. 394 (23 U.S.C. Sec. 794); 28 C.F.R. Secs. 41.56-.58.1988. Department of Justice, coordination of federal security, 504 access standards.

Statutory and regulatory standards often require changes in many components of an established center's operations—physical facility design, staff composition, admission and discharge policies, record-keeping practices, fee schedules, range of services offered, and participant reassessment procedures.

Previous Research

Few studies to date have addressed issues of regulation and quality standards in the home care industry (Schlenker et al., 1989), and none has focused on regulation in the adult day care industry. On the other hand, some findings of recent studies of the effects of licensure and certification on nursing home operations may be expected to apply to adult day care. Most of these studies have found that although licensure and certification requirements for health care providers are intended to ensure a minimally acceptable level of care to clients, legislated standards have not necessarily fostered this goal (Ruchlin, 1977, 1979; Pegels, 1980; Mahler, 1981; Grimaldi, 1984; Luft, 1985; Day & Klein, 1987). In other words, research has shown a wide gap between legislative intentions and legislative effects. Researchers have found three predominant causes for this gap: provider resistance to costs often incurred in meeting standards; the frequently confusing structure of the regulations; and poor coordination among administrating agencies.

Cost is perhaps the most fundamental issue. Ruchlin (1977) reported that regulation is often seen as counter to care providers' interests. Grimaldi (1984) agreed that the financial interests of providers cannot be ignored and noted that regulations that include incentives for providers seem to be more effective than those that do not. Grimaldi also suggested that future regulatory changes might rely on financial incentives to further public goals. Smits (1984) has cataloged some of the incentives and disincentives to socially desirable behavior inherent in alternative means of nursing home reimbursement.

Uncertainty on the part of day care staff about meeting costs of compliance and deciding on specific changes necessary under the requirements stems in large part from the often-confusing language in the regulations. As legislators adjust earlier miscalculations and address emerging needs, laws are necessarily constructed piecemeal. Thus, the nature of the legislative process itself contributes to the problem (Ruchlin, 1977; Mahler, 1981; Grimaldi, 1984; Luft, 1985). Grimaldi (1984), however, predicted that much of the confusion could be resolved within the next few years by several legislative changes including consolidation of Medicaid and Medicare certification requirements to eliminate differently phrased, but nearly identical, requirements in the regulations and elimination of duplicate standards and standards that do not affect quality.

Enforcement is the key to effective regulation. Pegels (1980) has pointed out that the lag time between legislation and its effective implementation is a problem. The most frequently cited impediment to enforcement, however, is the division of responsibility among various administrating agencies (Ruchlin, 1977, 1979; Mahler, 1981; Grimaldi, 1984). Mahler (1981) suggested that the large number of administrative agencies involved in health care regulation and the constraining requirements under which each agency must operate inhibit the coordination needed for effective regulatory enforcement.

Overall, these studies of nursing home regulation appear to promise mixed results from regulatory efforts. Commentators suggest that the regulatory effort may be unrelated to patient care, inimical to providers' interests, uncoordinated, loosely enforced, at times too vague while at other times too detailed, and often costly.

Nonetheless, regardless of the relative beneficial effects of regulation, Pegels (1980) suggested that the political trend is toward even tighter control in health care regulations. If he is right, states and funding sources can be expected to extend additional regulations to cover day care operations as demand for adult day care grows among the nation's elderly. Consequently, we sought to answer the following questions:

- What is the present scope of licensure and certification in the day care industry, and how similar are the requirements of these two types of regulation?
- To what extent have licensure and certification penetrated the adult day care industry?
- What differences, if any, are found between licensed and unlicensed and certified and uncertified centers?
- What are provider attitudes toward the necessity and perceived costs of regulation?

Data Collection and Methodology

Our data came from three sources: interviews with center directors, participant records, and state regulatory agencies. Statistically significant differences (e.g., between licensed and unlicensed centers, between certified and uncertified centers, and between Model I and Model II) were evaluated for categorical variables with χ^2 tests and with analysis of variance for continuous variables. To minimize the possibility of finding a significant difference from chance alone, pairwise comparisons were investigated only if the overall comparison was found to be significant. In all analyses, weights based on the sampling design were used.

As part of data collection, day care center directors were asked what specific changes in the operations or in the physical facility of the center were required to meet regulatory standards. The directors were also asked if they thought each change was necessary to ensure effective care and whether the change had affected costs.

In addition to center visits, we gathered data on the regulatory requirements for each of the 18 states (Alabama, Arizona, California, Connecticut, Kansas, Louisiana, Maine, Massachusetts, Maryland, Michigan, Minnesota, Mississippi, New York, South Carolina, Tennessee, Texas, Wisconsin, and the District of Columbia) in which sampled centers were located. This information came from telephone interviews with licensing and certification agencies and documents forwarded from them. More than two-thirds of these states licensed and/or certified adult day care centers.

Results

SCOPE OF REGULATION

In the absence of federal guidelines, licensing requirements commonly vary from state to state. Some similar requirements for both certification and licensure, however, affected center services, staff composition and numbers, facility characteristics, and hours of operation.

Service provision was usually regulated in terms of type of service(s) provided and sometimes in terms of the quality of the service. While Birnbaum reported that services covered under Title XX of the Social Security Act (the Social Services Block Grant) vary by state, services usually include "social work evaluation and counseling, recreational activities . . . the preparation and serving of food, transportation, educational and training activities" (Birnbaum, 1981, p. 96). Palmer (1985) reported that services provided under the Massachusetts Medicaid day care program followed directly from stated system objectives: provision of therapeutic recreation and services, social services and counseling, personal care, and necessary transportation; restoration of health; and assistance with adequate nutrition.

California's service requirements were similar. Harder et al. (1986) reported that the state Adult Day Health Care Act of 1978 and MediCal legislation allowed California to become one of the first states to "offer this outpatient alternative to institutional long-term care as a mandated Medicaid benefit" (Harder et al., 1986, p. 429). Services in these programs (adult day health centers, ADHCs) included medical and therapeutic efforts as well as personal care assistance.

According to Kurland (1982), New Jersey required provision of eight basic services for a medical day care center to receive state funds: "medical, nursing, social services, transportation, personal care, dietary, social activities, and rehabilitative services" (p. 48). Occupational therapy was included under the state's per diem reimbursement rate, while physical and speech therapies required an additional approval process for funding.

Nutritional services are addressed by both licensing and certification regulations. They usually specify nutritional quality (percentage of recommended daily allowance, RDA) and amount of food provided to participants. California's nutritional standards are typical. Licensing requirements of the California Department of Health Services stipulate that an adult day care participant attending for four hours must be served one meal that provides one-third of the RDA. A participant who attends for eight hours must receive either one meal plus snacks or two meals and snacks that equal one-half of the RDA. Certification standards of the California State MediCal Assistance Program are identical.

Regulations of licensing as well as certifying agencies often affect center staffing. The number of required staff members is generally determined by specified staff-to-participant ratios that range from as low as 1:5.1 to as high as 1:25.1. Some guidelines allow for flexibility. The Kansas Department of Social and Rehabilitation Services' licensing regulations, for example, specify a ratio of 1:12 when services are being provided and allow a higher ratio of 1:15 when participants are in the center but are not receiving services.

Licensing and certification regulations also commonly specify certain administrative and caregiving positions, often including the skill level of the staff. Most require a full-time director and at least one other staff member (often a nurse) and dictate training and experience required for individuals who fill these positions. Regulations generally require a bachelor's degree and from one to three years of experience for both positions, although some licensing and certification criteria allow substitution of experience for the degree. The center director's job is usually specified as full time, although time could be shared among the day care center and other affiliated agency functions.

Few licensing or certification criteria address the number of aides, and specifications for nursing requirements vary. Most regulatory policies, however, do require a registered nurse (RN) or RN supervisor.

In addition to staffing and service requirements, both licensure and certification regulations may affect physical facilities in terms of total physical space that must be available for the participant population in the aggregate, space per participant, number of bathroom facilities, barrier-free access, and fire exits. A center applying for licensure and certification frequently must undertake alterations in its facility to qualify (see the following discussion).

Most states also require that at a minimum a written record be kept for each participant, but only a few stipulate record content.

The Extent of Regulation

LICENSURE

Licensing requirements vary from state to state, and some affect only particular types of day care services, allowing centers to hold more than one license if they provide more than one health care service. Additionally, governing bodies often allow the affiliated, or parent, organizations license to cover the day care component (Von Behren, 1986).

Consistent with previous findings (Von Behren, 1986), just over half of the centers studied reported holding at least one license (Table 4.1). In general centers were licensed as either adult day health centers or social or nonspecific adult day care centers. A small percentage of the centers held multiple licenses in one of four combinations: (1) adult day health and social or nonspecific adult day care; (2) adult day health and outpatient

Table 4.1
Program Licensure Characteristics by Model

	Overall (*n* = 45)	Model I (*n* = 13)	Model II (*n* = 28)	Special (*n* = 4)
Percentage licensed	53.9%	34.0%	74.9%	12.1%
Type of license held				
Adult day health	56.4	100.0	47.5	0.0
Social or nonspecific	40.8	0.0	52.7	0.0
Outpatient rehabilitation	2.9	15.0	0.0	0.0
Day treatment	2.9	0.0	0.0	100.0
Other	11.1	0.0	14.3	0.0
Licensing agency				
State health department	70.5	100.0	63.3	0.0
County/local health	15.9	0.0	22.9	0.0
State social/service	9.6	0.0	13.8	0.0
Mental health agency	4.0	0.0	0.0	100.0

Note: Programs may hold more than one type of license.

rehabilitation; (3) adult day health and other; and (4) social or nonspecific adult day care and other.

Standards varied by type of license, usually requiring more rigorous standards for health-related licensure than for social or nonspecific licensure. The licensing agency for most licensed centers was the state health department.

One of our interests was whether or not centers in our three models differed in their licensure status. We found that while Model II centers were in general more likely than either Model I or Special Purpose centers to be licensed, they were less likely than Model I centers to be licensed as an adult day health center. In fact, all the licensed Model I centers were licensed as an adult day health center, compared to less than half of the licensed Model II centers. Model II centers, on the other hand, often were more likely to be licensed as nonspecific adult day care centers (see Table 4.1).

CERTIFICATION

Certification can be required for a number of types of funding (usually federal), most often Medicaid and Medicare but also Social Services Block Grant and Older Americans Act funding. Just over half of the centers studied were certified, and an additional 13 percent reported plans to apply for certification in the next year. At the time of the survey, 40 percent of the centers were both licensed and certified, and 33 percent were neither licensed nor certified.

Table 4.2 shows what funds the centers were certified to receive and identifies the certifying agencies. The most common funding source for the sample centers that were certified was Medicaid. Many of the centers in the sample were certified for multiple funding sources, although the state Medicaid office was the most frequent certifying agency.

Table 4.2 also shows the percentage of Model I, Model II, and Special Purpose centers certified for each funding source. Consistent with findings in the finance chapter (i.e., Model II centers receive more Medicaid and other public funds, while Model I centers are more dependent on private monies), Model II programs were more likely to be certified to receive Medicaid funds.

Differences between Regulated and Unregulated Centers

Tables 4.3 through 4.7 compare licensed and unlicensed and certified and uncertified centers. We compared center characteristics in five domains: staffing, services, facility, attendance, and participants. In general, regu-

Table 4.2
Program Certification by Model

	Overall (n = 45)	Model I (n = 13)	Model II (n = 28)	Special (n = 4)
Percentage certified	53.5%	50.1%	60.6%	21.1%
Plan to apply for certification	13.0	0.0	16.0	0.0
Funding source				
Medicaid	78.1	47.7	89.8	100.0
Title XX	27.8	52.3	18.6	57.1
Aging office	17.7	52.3	4.2	0.0
Medicare	2.9	12.7	0.0	0.0
Other state	2.9	0.0	4.2	0.0
State Medicaid	53.9	47.7	57.9	57.1
State social security	29.4	52.3	21.0	57.1
State health office	17.5	0.0	21.1	57.1
State mental health association	2.2	0.0	0.0	42.9
Other	2.8	0.0	0.0	57.1

Note: Programs may be certified for more than one funding source and by more than one agency.

lated centers differed from their unregulated counterparts, suggesting that regulation probably does affect the industry. Despite the limitations of small sample sizes at the center level, many of the comparisons were statistically significant.

Although some differences were small and not always in the expected direction, data in the tables suggested that:

- Regulated centers differed from unregulated centers in each of the five domains compared;
- Differences were somewhat more likely to occur between certified and uncertified centers than between licensed and unlicensed centers;
- The magnitude of differences associated with licensure was about the same as that associated with certification.

Staffing differences were more apparent between certified and uncertified centers than between licensed and unlicensed centers (Table 4.3). Certified centers had more staff as well as more skilled staff per participant. They were more likely than uncertified centers to employ a medical director, as well as a registered nurse. In addition, while no differences were apparent in staffing ratios between licensed and unlicensed centers,

Table 4.3
Staffing Characteristics by Licensure and Certification Status

Characteristic	Overall	Licensed	Unlicensed	Certified	Uncertified
Percentage employing:					
Medical director	51	54	48	64+	37+
Registered nurse	69	68	65	77	52
RN or LPN	75	77	65	53	56
Social worker	51	43	53	57	33
Staff-to-participant ratios:					
All staff	1:2.9	1:2.9	1:30	1:2.6+	1:4.7+
RN or LPN	1:33.3	1:29.3	1:29.5	1:19.7+	1:74.1+
Aides	1:12.5	1:11.7	1:12.5	1:10.5	1:15.3
Administrative	1:12.5	1:11.1	1:12.8	1:11.2	1:13.2

Note: Data include only paid staff.
+Indicates that pairwise comparison is significant ($p < .05$).

certified centers had a significantly higher staff-to-participant ratio than did uncertified centers, and a significantly higher nurse-to-participant ratio than uncertified centers.

Both certified and licensed centers were also more likely than their unregulated counterparts to offer any given service (Table 4.4). They were more likely to provide transportation, case management, and a variety of professional and other services. Bathing was an exception: unregulated centers were more likely than their regulated centers to offer bathing. This is probably because unlicensed and uncertified centers often were housed in an inpatient facility with bathing facilities.

The primary difference in facilities between regulated and unregulated centers was that certified or licensed centers were more often housed in buildings that were solely used for day care (Table 4.5). Additionally, if a center was regulated it was more likely than an unregulated one to meet 504 standards for handicap access. Health inspections, on the other hand, did not appear to depend on being regulated, while fire inspection was more likely to occur in unregulated centers.

Regulation also was associated with variations in attendance patterns (Table 4.6). Regulated centers served more participants each day; they were more likely to have a waiting list, and their participants attended more frequently per week. These differences may reflect either a response to the enhanced availability of services in regulated centers, or, more likely, publicly subsidized participants simply were more likely to attend regulated than nonregulated centers.

Table 4.4
Service Provision by Licensure and Certification Status

Characteristic	Overall	Licensed	Unlicensed	Certified	Uncertified
Nursing	81%	87%	75%	98% +	65% +
Medical supervision	80	86	75	96 +	65 +
Case management	71	90 +	52 +	77	65
Nutrition education	67	87 +	48 +	70	64
Transportation	64	89 +	39 +	76	52
Physical therapy	42	43	41	46	39
Breakfast	32	28	36	36	29
Shopping	29	43	16	28	31
Bathing	29	10 +	50 +	23	36
Occupational therapy	26	24	29	27	26
Physician	21	35 +	6 +	31	10
Drug consultation	15	23	6	25	4

+ Indicates that pairwise comparison is significant ($p < .05$).

Table 4.7 illustrates the case-mix differences between licensed and unlicensed and certified and uncertified centers. Participants of regulated centers generally were younger, more often were female, unmarried, and from a minority group, and more often publicly subsidized.

Provider Attitudes toward
the Necessity and Costs of Regulation

Licensing and certification standards required centers to make changes in physical facilities, staffing composition and numbers, admissions and discharge policies, record keeping, fee schedules, and participant reassessment procedures. Table 4.8 shows the percentage of centers that made these changes. Also shown are the reported opinions of the center directors concerning whether the change was necessary or unnecessary (to meet operating standards outside of the regulatory requirements), and whether it affected program cost.

Almost one-third of the directors reported that adjustments to their center's physical facility were required to comply with regulatory standards. Most were made in response to Medicaid or Social Services Block Grant requirements. Almost all these changes were perceived as necessary, and only a very small percentage of the changes related to accessibility, fire and

Table 4.5
Facility Characteristics by Licensure and Certification Status

Characteristic	Overall	Licensed	Unlicensed	Certified	Uncertified
Building only for adult day care	17%	33% +	3% +	29%	5%
504 standards	88	97	78	100 +	75 +
Health inspection	68	58	77	77	58
Fire inspection	97	94	100	94	100

+ Indicates that pairwise comparison is significant ($p < .05$).

safety, and size were perceived as affecting cost. (However, other types of changes to the physical facility were all perceived as affecting costs.)

Changes in staff numbers and composition were also frequently required, and in this case they were typically perceived as affecting program cost. However, as with the facility changes, most center directors felt they were necessary.

Adjustments in admissions and discharge policies were also typically required and judged to be necessary, even though some were perceived to have affected program costs. Record-keeping practices were also frequently affected by regulatory requirements. Nearly one-fourth of each of the required changes in centers' record-keeping procedures were perceived to have affected costs, but most directors of these centers felt that the changes were necessary.

Directors also generally approved of required changes in fee schedules and increases in the frequency of participant reassessment.

Table 4.6
Attendance Patterns by Licensure and Certification Status

Characteristic	Overall	Licensed	Unlicensed	Certified	Uncertified
Average daily census (participants)	18	22 +	15 +	21 +	16 +
Waiting list (percent)	30	46 +	13 +	41	17
Program age (years)	5.4	6.1	4.8	5.5	5.3
Average days/week	3.4	3.9	3.0	3.8	3.1

+ Indicates that pairwise comparison is significant ($p < .05$).

Table 4.7
Center's Aggregate Participant Characteristics by Licensure and Certification Status

Characteristic	Overall	Licensed	Unlicensed	Certified	Uncertified
Medicaid reimbursement	26	45 +	6 +	45 +	7 +
Title XX reimbursement	16	26 +	6 +	16	17
Private pay only	34	17 +	53 +	24 +	45 +
SSI recipients	19	30 +	9 +	29 +	10 +
Over 85	18	11 +	24 +	16	19
Male	42	31 +	53 +	38	46
Married	31	23 +	39 +	26	36
White	68	57 +	80 +	63	73
Mental disorders	39	37	42	38	41
No ADL dependencies	42	47	37	42	43
Average number ADLs	1.7	1.6	1.8	1.8	1.6
Average number IADLs	1.8	2.1	1.5	1.8	1.8

Note: All numbers are percentages unless otherwise specified. ADL, activity of daily living; IADL, instrumental activity of daily living.
+ Indicates that pairwise comparison is significant ($p < .05$).

Conclusions

Results of this national survey showed that licensing and certification regulations were quite similar in their requirements and touched nearly all phases of adult day care operations: staffing composition and numbers, service provision, physical facilities, record keeping, and administrative and caregiving policies and procedures.

The regulations often were perceived by center directors as having required changes in many or most of these components of the operations of established centers. Consistent with these perceptions, regulated centers differed from their unregulated counterparts in the following ways:

- Certified centers were more likely to employ more skilled and more staff per participant;
- Both certified and licensed centers were more likely to offer various services;

– 75 –

- Regulated centers were more likely to be housed in facilities that met 504 standards and were used exclusively for day care;
- Regulated centers served participants who attended more frequently and in larger numbers;
- Regulated centers served participants who were more likely to be publicly subsidized, racial minorities, unmarried, and younger.

In the opinion of the center directors, one of the most common and costly changes required for regulatory compliance was in staff composition and number: licensure and certification standards addressed both staff-to-participant ratios and skill mix.

These findings suggested that both licensure and certification probably do affect day care center operations. Making the appropriate changes is likely to involve some costs, but centers that make the changes and acquire licensure or certification often are rewarded with a larger census, probably because publicly subsidized participants are more likely to be placed in licensed and certified centers.

Whether or not participant outcomes are affected by structural consequences of regulation was beyond the scope of this study.

Table 4.8
Changes Required by Licensing or Certification Standards and Program Directors'
Reported Opinions Concerning Necessity of Change and Effects on Program Costs

Change	Directors' opinions: percentage who said regulation		
	Affected programs	Were necessary	Affected cost
Physical Facility			
Accessibility	30.1	90.7	5.1
Fire and safety	32.8	91.4	4.7
Size	30.1	100.0	5.1
Other	14.2	80.2	100.0
Staffing			
Number employed	45.5	91.8	78.0
Composition	52.3	93.2	70.1
Other	8.4	100.0	100.0
Policies			
Admission criteria	37.2	100.0	11.7
Discharge criteria	21.3	100.0	20.5
Establish or expand written policies	30.5	100.0	14.3
Other	11.4	100.0	100.0
Record Keeping			
Initiate participant care plans	36.2	92.2	28.0
Addition/changes to participant records	38.4	92.7	26.4
Service delivery	35.7	92.1	28.4
Fiscal record keeping	45.3	100.0	22.4
Other	15.2	100.0	26.1
Quality of Care			
Frequency and measurement	25.4	88.9	39.8
Care review process	28.1	100.0	36.0
Record audits	38.5	100.0	26.3
Other	2.8	100.0	100.0
Financial Matters			
Charge/fee schedule	48.3	100.0	31.8
Budgeting process	24.1	100.0	42.1
Accounting method	34.8	91.9	29.1
Other	2.8	100.0	100.0

FIVE

FINANCIAL ASPECTS OF
ADULT DAY CARE

CURRENT and complete financial information is crucial to making informed decisions about the expansion of adult day care. Although several focused studies have been undertaken, the last comprehensive examination of the financial aspects of adult day care was conducted in the mid-1970s (Weissert, 1976).

This chapter updates existing information on both revenues and expenses of the growing adult day care industry. Two questions guided the data collection and analyses: How are adult day care centers in the United States currently funded? What are the major operating expenses of adult day care centers? In the Results section, we present a financial profile of the adult day care industry, describe the key components of unit costs, and discuss the possible effects of capacity utilization on the survey findings.

Previous Research

Studies addressing the financial aspects of adult day care that have been published since 1970 include works by Novick (1973), Weissert (1975, 1976, 1978), Weiler et al. (1976), Weiler & Rathbone-McCuan (1978), Weissert et al. (1980), Sands & Suzuki (1983), Hannan & O'Donnell (1984), Mace & Rabins (1984), and Von Behren (1986).

REVENUE SOURCES

Previous research shows that funding for adult day care comes from a variety of public and private sources. At the federal and state levels, funds are available from Medicaid, Social Services Block Grants, and Older Americans Act monies. Medicare does not reimburse for day care per se; instead, reimbursement is for specific rehabilitative therapies and is often funneled through a certified Medicare outpatient affiliate. Other sources of financing include private fees and donations, local government monies, and foundations. Weissert (1975, 1976), in his study of 10 day care centers, found that centers affiliated with general hospitals or social service agencies were less likely to qualify for the service-specific funding associated with Medicare, but did receive Medicaid, Social Services Block Grant, and Older Americans Act (OAA)–Title III funding.

A national survey of adult day care centers conducted by the National Institute of Adult Daycare (NIAD) found that Medicaid provided the largest source of funds for the industry, and participant fees were the second major source (Von Behren, 1986). In a report describing the Harbor Area Adult Daycare center in California, Sands & Suzuki (1983) reported that direct fees provided the largest source of funds for the center (47 percent), while foundation, organizational, and individual donations constituted just over one-fourth of centers' funding.

An example of local government funding is provided by Weiler et al. (1976) and Weiler & Rathbone-McCuan (1978) in their reports on the Lexington, Kentucky Center for Creative Living, which was funded in part by the local health department.

COSTS

Weissert (1975, 1976) found the mean cost per participant day to be $25.09; the daily cost ranged from $11.26 to $61.56, although most centers fell within a fairly narrow range close to the median of $21.32. Sands & Suzuki (1983) reported the 1981 cost per participant day at the Harbor Area Adult Daycare Center to be $23.35. In a national survey of day care centers serving clients with Alzheimer's disease, Mace & Rabins (1984) found that the mean cost per participant day was $21.32, with a range of $0 to $55.00 per day. The NIAD national survey found an annual average center budget was $137,085, and the average per diem cost was $31, with a median of $20 (Von Behren, 1986). When in-kind contributions were excluded from these calculations, the average cost dropped to $27 per participant day.

Increased operating costs have been found to be associated with service intensity. Weissert (1975, 1976) found that Model I (nursing and therapeutically oriented) centers were generally more costly than social interaction-oriented centers. Weissert also found that per diem costs were higher in Model I than in Model II (social interaction-oriented) centers, an average of $20 and $40, respectively; the highest per diem health service was nursing care, and the highest per diem support service was participant supervision. Hannan & O'Donnell (1984), in a study of 15 New York State centers, found that direct cost per hour increased as the level of ancillary services increased. Among Hannan and O'Donnell's three categories of centers (support, mixed, and ancillary; in which the support category closely mirrors Weissert's Model I, and the ancillary closely mirrors Model II), ancillary centers were found to be the most costly. Hannan & O'Donnell reported that medical and therapeutic care were the most expensive services. Mace & Rabins (1984) found higher costs to be associated with the provision of professional services.

The composition of a center's staff also affects costs of day care. Weissert (1978) found nursing homes and adult day care centers to be quite similar in terms of total staff numbers in relation to participant populations, but day care centers employed more expensive, skilled personnel and a larger number of administrators.

In terms of specific services, bus transportation was the highest operational expenses (excluding salaries) in Novick's (1973) list of expenses for the day hospital center at Maimondes Hospital and Home for the Aged in Montreal, Canada. Transportation was also a high-cost service in Weissert's (1975, 1976) sample centers, and Mace & Rabins (1984) found that centers that owned or leased a bus tended to report higher costs.

Weiler et al. (1976) found meals to be the most expensive service item at the Lexington, Kentucky Center for Creative Living; the high cost was caused in part by the large amount of staff time spent serving meals. At the Lexington center most services were provided through contract, and total cost per participant day was $12.99, which included $4.22 for meals, $3.62 for health services, $2.62 for recreation, and $2.53 for transportation.

NET INCOME

Mace and Rabins (1984) reported that 48 percent of the centers studied reported that they were breaking even and that centers that had been in operation for less than six years were less likely to be breaking even. Novick (1973) indicated that the day hospital center at Maimondes was operating at an annual loss that was partly defrayed by auxiliary contributions. Sands & Suzuki (1983) reported that The Harbor Area Adult Daycare center received community help to make up the difference between private pay fees and true costs.

DATA COLLECTION

Survey data were collected between July 1, 1985, and September 30, 1986. (For a comprehensive description of the methodology and data collection, see Chapter 1). Initial financial data were gathered during the first collection phase in which 12 sites (which themselves constituted a random subsample) were contacted by telephone. Following the telephone contact, teams of two persons visited each site for two days. The teams collected center data and attempted to gather financial data for the last five years of the center's operations. These efforts to collect detailed financial data revealed four problems: (1) most sites could furnish only data concerning their most recent fiscal year; (2) a number of sites did not have audited financial data; (3) data consistency among sites, and within a site over time, varied considerably as a result of differential funding source requirements, record-keeping procedures, and center modifications; and (4) only a few sites could furnish full-accrual data.

Because of these problems, data collection procedures were adjusted for the remaining 48 sites. Data collection forms were mailed in advance to the sample centers. These mailings were following by one-day/one-person site visits and subsequent telephone calls to assist center personnel in completing the forms. Returned forms were checked for reliability and completeness, and follow-up questions were sent to sites for clarification or modification. After the forms were again returned to the research team, they were checked for completeness and reliability a second time. Finally, when necessary, telephone follow-up helped to complete the data set.

DATA ANALYSIS

Given the diversity of accounting and reporting procedures among the sites, we implemented a two-step process to make the data comparable. First, because reported data represented a center's latest fiscal year, data covered a 36-month period: January 1983 to December 1986. Thus, month-by-month adjustments, using the Consumer Price Index detailed report and the Employment Cost Index, were made to bring the data into conformity with the fiscal year beginning July 1, 1985. Data for the nine sites whose reported fiscal year began after July 1, 1985, were adjusted backward, and the sites whose reported fiscal year began before July 1 were adjusted forward so that their fiscal year began July 1, 1985.

Second, for each site that reported an in-kind revenue or an in-kind expense, we checked to ensure that their reported in-kind revenues equaled their reported in-kind expenses. If in-kind revenues and expenses did not match they were adjusted to reflect full-accrual accounting procedures.

Data were analyzed in total and in two auspice models. Results for Special Purpose centers are omitted because the number of these sites reporting complete fiscal information was judged to be too small for meaningful conclusions. Medians instead of means are reported because of sample size and, in some cases, skewed data.

Despite the extensive efforts discussed here, complete revenue, expense, and staffing data were available for only 31 centers. Thus, care should be taken in generalizing outside of the sample. However, the sites for which complete fiscal data were available did not differ significantly from the remainder of the sample in terms of average daily census; percentage of participants dependent, over age 65, or receiving Medicaid funding; or provision of a transportation service. The sites reporting complete financial data were, however, significantly ($p < .05$) more likely to employ a licensed practical or registered nurse. In addition, they were significantly more likely to be located in the West (where centers tend not to be licensed, but tend to be certified) and were less likely to be located in the Northeast.

Results are reported in three sections: (1) industry analysis of revenues, expenses, and profits; (2) unit analysis of revenues and costs; and (3) capacity adjustments. The first section provides an overview of the industry as a whole, and the second section focuses on revenues and costs per participant day. The third section, capacity adjustments, presents an exploratory analysis concerning efficient operations.

Revenues, Expenses, and Profits

MEDIAN REVENUES

The median annual revenue of the sites reporting full fiscal data was $143,660. A quarter of the sites have revenues below $103,436, while another quarter had revenues above $179,391. Auspice Model I sites ($61,958) had a lower median revenue than Auspice Model II sites ($123,278), as well as a wider distribution of reported revenues.

REVENUE SOURCES

More than half of all centers reported the receipt of revenue from self-pay per diem, private non–per diem funds, and Medicaid. Other common sources of revenue were in-kind contributions, Older Americans Act funds, fund raising, and Social Services Block Grant monies, as well as monies from foundations (Table 5.1).

Although more than half of all centers received Medicaid funds, only a small percentage of centers (2.4 percent) reported receipt of Medicare funds (see Table 5.1).

About half of reported revenues (47.5 percent) were from federal agencies, and more than one-fourth were from nongovernmental sources (Table 5.2). Medicaid was the largest single source of funds, accounting for more than one-fourth of all the revenues received by the industry. The second highest percentage of funding came from private (non–per diem) sources (16.6 percent), which included monetary and nonmonetary bequests and donations from participants, participants' families, and private citizens. These sources were followed by self-pay (per diem), which constituted 15.6 percent of all revenues received. The remaining major fund-

Table 5.1
Percentage of Centers Receiving Funds by Source and Model

Source	Percentage receiving funds		
	All sites ($n = 32$)	Model I ($n = 9$)	Model II ($n = 23$)
Federal			
Medicaid	55.9	38.8	63.0
Older American Act	39.6	33.5	42.2
Social Services Block Grant	20.7	8.2	25.9
Medicare	2.4	8.2	0.0
Other	9.7	0.0	13.7
Any Federal	87.1	80.4	89.8
Nongovernmental			
Private (non per diem)	52.0	24.5	63.5
In kind, other	46.9	55.6	34.9
United Way	15.7	8.2	18.8
Private religious	4.7	0.0	6.6
Outside foundation	4.7	8.2	3.2
Fundraising	26.3	11.7	32.3
Own foundation	18.1	0.0	25.6
Sponsor	2.3	0.0	3.2
Any nongovermental	87.9	91.8	86.3
Self-Pay (per diem)	58.3	67.4	54.6
Nonfederal Governmental			
Other public	20.7	17.9	21.9
State monies	9.7	0.0	13.7
Local monies	4.8	0.0	6.8
Any nonfederal governmental	32.8	26.0	35.6

ing sources included: Older Americans Act monies (10.5 percent); Social Services Block Grant (7.8 percent); and in-kind contributions (5.2 percent).

Revenue sources differed regionally. Centers in the Northeast were the most dependent on per diem funding. For centers in the Northeast, per diem funding accounted for more than one-third (39.6 percent) of all funds; in the North Central (11.1 percent), South (8.8 percent), and West (2.3 percent), a considerably smaller proportion of funds was received as per diem payments.

Table 5.2
Industry Revenues by Source and Model

| | Percentage of total funds received | | |
Source	All sites (n = 32)	Model I (n = 9)	Model II (n = 23)
Federal			
Medicaid	26.8	12.4	33.5
Older American Act	10.5	3.6	13.7
Social Services Block Grant	7.8	1.9	10.6
Medicare	1.5	4.9	0.0
Other	0.9	0.0	1.3
Subtotal	47.5	22.8	59.1
Nongovernmental			
Private (non per diem)	16.6	44.8	3.6
In kind, other	5.2	3.9	5.8
United Way	2.4	0.1	3.5
Private religious	1.7	0.0	2.4
Outside foundation	1.1	2.4	0.6
Fundraising	0.2	0.0	0.3
Own foundation	0.1	0.0	0.2
Sponsor	0.1	0.0	0.2
Subtotal	27.4	51.2	16.6
Self-Pay (per diem)	15.6	15.6	15.6
Nonfederal Governmental			
Other public	4.8	4.4	5.0
State	4.0	6.0	3.1
Local	0.6	0.0	0.8
Subtotal	9.4	10.4	8.9
Total	100	100	100

Sources of revenue also varied significantly between the two auspice models. Auspice Model I centers received just under half of their revenues from private (non–per diem) sources, with self-pay (per diem) accounting for the second largest proportion (15.6 percent) and Medicaid accounting for almost as much (12.4 percent). In contrast, Auspice Model II centers received their largest proportion of funding from Medicaid (33.3 percent), with self-pay (per diem), Older Americans Act, and Social Services Block Grant funds providing their next largest amount of funding (see Table 5.2).

Day care costs can be divided into two general categories—direct costs that include operational expenses for personnel, equipment, and supplies, and facilities used in providing services and indirect costs that include overhead. In-kind contributions such as volunteer services, donated supplies, and loaned equipment or facilities may be classified as either direct or indirect costs.

Table 5.3 provides an industry profile showing how centers spent their funds. Direct labor accounted for slightly more than half of total operating expenses (54.5 percent) and was the largest expense category for centers. The second most expensive item was transportation (12.2 percent), followed by facility expenses (10.5 percent), food costs (7.5 percent), and administrative costs (5.1 percent). Other expenses (which in aggregate accounted for less than 6 percent of the total expenses) included such items as utilities, programming, and development costs. Of the total reported expenses, 93 percent were actual expenses, while 7 percent were in-kind.

Table 5.4 shows median net income figures for our sample centers. The median net income for all sites was a loss of $1,815, with Auspice Model I

Table 5.3
Summary of Industry Expenses

	Percentage of total expenditures	Percentage of line item which is in kind
Labor	54.4	2.4
Transportation	12.2	5.2
Facility	10.5	29.6
Food	7.5	20.3
Administration	5.1	3.9
Other	5.5	5.2
Total direct	95.2	7.4
Allocated	4.8	
Total	100.0	11.9

Table 5.4
Median Profit and Product Margin[a] by Model

	Overall	Model I	Model II
Total revenue	$143,660	$100,908	$145,700
Total expenses	145,774	101,660	148,268
Avoidable expenses	133,999	101,660	141,205
Net income[b]	(1,815)	10,735	(3,171)
Profit margin percentage[c]	− 1.24	9.55	− 2.95
Product margin[d]	9,345	10,735	8,604
Product margin percentage[e]	6.12	9.55	5.52

[a]Figures are reported using accrual basis of accounting. Results did not differ significantly from results using cash basis of accounting.
[b]Total revenue minus total expenses.
[c]Net income divided by total revenue.
[d]Total revenue minus avoidable expenses.
[e]Product margin divided by total revenue.

sites showing a median net income of $10,735 and Auspice Model II sites showing a median net loss of $3,171. The median profit margin was a loss of 1.24 percent. When allocated (indirect) costs are excluded, the median profit margin (called "product margin") is 6.12 percent. Examination of these data on a cash basis yields similar results. This indicates that day care centers may have little latitude in making major operating changes or responding to exigencies in their environment.

Unit Revenues and Costs

REVENUES

Table 5.5 shows median and quartile revenues per participant day by revenue source and auspice model. The median for all sites was $28.82, with the medians for Auspice Model I and Auspice Model II centers being nearly equal. However, wide variation exists around these numbers, especially for Auspice Model I sites.

COSTS

The previous expense analysis provides a financial profile of the adult day care industry as a whole, but it does not address the costs of serving adult day care participants at the center level. This section focuses on the unit costs of day care, or the cost per participant per day. Five major cost items were examined: (1) total cost per participant day; (2) direct labor costs per participant day; (3) transportation costs per participant day; (4) facility costs per participant day; and (5) food costs per participant day. Combined costs for labor, transportation, facility, and food accounted for approximately three-fourths of a center's total expenses. Costs per participant day were derived by dividing the reported annual cost by the reported number of annual participant days.

TOTAL COST PER PARTICIPANT DAY

Table 5.6 shows median expense by cost category and by auspice model. The median total cost per participant day was $29.50. Although wide variation existed around the median, one-half of the sites had a cost between $23.40 and $36.10. There was little difference in the cost per participant day between Auspice Model I and Auspice Model II centers. When in-kind expenses are not included in the calculated cost per participant day, the median total cost drops from $29.50 to $25.20 per participant day.

DIRECT LABOR COSTS

The major component of the daily participant cost, direct labor, was approximately four times as expensive as the next largest cost component, transportation. In these analyses, direct labor was defined as labor provided either by center staff or through contractual services that did not overlap with transportation, food, facilities, or administrative costs. For example, direct labor included physical therapy or physicians' services, but excluded labor purchased in conjunction with meals and transportation services.

Most staff members were paid employees. The services of a physician or therapist tended to be provided by a consultant agreement, while in-kind staffing was usually for fiscal manager or bookkeeping services.

The median direct labor cost was $14.60 per participant day. Centers at the 75th percentile had a direct labor cost per participant day of $22.80, while those at the 25th percentile had a cost of $10.30. Labor costs varied significantly between Auspice Model I and Auspice Model II centers. Auspice Model I centers had a median direct labor cost per participant day of $22.80, approximately 60 percent higher than the $14.20 median cost for Auspice Model II centers. This difference results at least partially from the significantly higher average staff-to-participant ratio found among Auspice Model I centers. (These figures should be interpreted with care because of the large variation around the medians, especially among Auspice Model I sites.)

Table 5.5
Median and Quartile Revenues per Participant Day by Source and Model

Source	Median amount received			Bottom quartile			Top quartile		
	All sites (n = 29)	Model I (n = 8)	Model II (n = 21)	All sites	Model I	Model II	All sites	Model I	Model II
Federal									
Medicaid	$15.11	$13.87	$16.21	$10.06	$7.69	$9.87	$23.53	$18.10	$25.82
Older American Act	2.61	7.88	2.56	2.12	7.88	2.04	8.96	7.88	9.48
Social Services block grant	9.87	12.82	8.96	7.45	12.82	5.93	13.32	12.82	17.73
Medicare	21.59	21.59	—	21.59	21.59	—	21.59	21.59	—
Other	0.70	—	0.70	0.56	—	0.56	2.67	—	2.67
Subtotal	$17.62	$13.87	$20.95	$13.12	$12.82	$13.30	$25.79	$22.06	$28.26
Nongovernmental									
Private (non per diem)	$0.37	$39.27	$0.30	$0.14	$8.94	$0.12	$1.82	$180.96	$0.55
In kind, other	3.20	3.94	3.12	1.08	1.08	0.80	4.31	10.34	4.03

United Way	3.49	0.50	4.74	1.26	0.50	2.38	6.73	7.09
Private religious	2.06	—	2.06	0.09	—	0.09	13.49	13.49
Outside foundation	10.33	14.72	5.94	5.94	14.72	5.94	14.72	5.94
Fundraising	0.15	0.14	0.22	0.14	0.14	0.13	0.32	0.33
Own foundation	0.16	—	0.16	0.08	—	0.05	0.17	0.17
Sponsor	1.65	—	1.65	1.65	—	1.65	1.65	1.65
Subtotal	$3.51	$14.26	$2.14	$0.45	$1.96	$0.31	$12.59	$6.70
Self-Pay (per diem)	$5.12	$10.30	$3.33	$1.00	$4.91	$0.34	$12.41	$10.87
Nonfederal Governmental								
Other public	$7.21	$10.45	$5.05	$4.16	$7.96	$3.98	$10.48	$9.00
State	8.89	19.14	5.04	1.20	19.14	1.20	19.14	8.89
Local	2.80	—	2.80	2.21	—	2.21	3.39	3.39
Subtotal	$8.42	$12.94	$5.05	$4.07	$7.96	$3.70	$11.63	$9.81
Total	$28.82	$29.21	$28.42	$25.56	$24.16	$21.99	$34.61	$31.89

Note: Each figure includes only sites that reported revenues >$0.00. The subtotals and total represent the median subtotals and total revenues per participant day over all included sites, not the sum of the component categories.

Table 5.6
Median Expense by Cost Category and Model of Day Care

	All sites	Model I	Model II
Total Cost			
Median	$29.50	$31.20	$29.20
25th[a]	23.40	26.40	18.60
75th[a]	36.10	71.00	35.10
Labor			
Median	14.60	22.80	14.20
25th	10.30	11.60	8.90
75th	22.80	51.10	18.30
Transportation			
Median	3.30	4.00	3.10
25th	1.90	0.50	1.90
75th	4.50	6.90	4.20
Facility			
Median	2.70	5.20	2.60
25th	1.20	1.90	1.20
75th	4.70	9.40	3.20
Food			
Median	2.40	2.50	1.80
25th	0.80	2.40	0.50
75th	2.80	5.20	2.70
Allocated			
Median	0.00	0.00	0.00
25th	0.00	0.00	0.00
75th	2.70	0.70	3.60
Administrative			
Median	1.00	0.00	1.20
25th	0.50	0.00	0.60
75th	1.60	1.00	2.20

Note: Components do not sum to total median costs because reported component costs
are medians.
[a]Percentile.

TRANSPORTATION COSTS

Transportation was the second-largest component of cost per participant day. Transportation costs are those incurred in providing transportation services either to and from the center or for field trips, medical appointments, and errands. They include costs such as vehicle maintenance, labor, and gas. Most of the centers that offered transportation provided it themselves (68 percent), but some provided it through contract (18.7 percent), and others provided some transportation services and purchased the rest (13.1 percent).

For all sites reporting fiscal data, the median transportation cost per participant day was $3.30 (see Table 5.6). Half the centers incurred transportation costs per participant day between $1.90 and $4.50. When only those sites that provided a transportation service (27 of 29) were included in the analysis, the median transportation cost rose to $3.85 per participant day. Transportation costs per participant did not differ significantly between the two models.

FACILITY COSTS

Facility costs were the third-largest component of cost per participant day. These costs included rent or mortgage; any regular payments that covered the cost of occupying primary center space; housekeeping and general facility maintenance; major repairs or renovations; and labor directly related to these expenses.

The median facility cost per participant day across all sites was $2.70 (Table 5.6). One quarter had a facilities cost per participant day less than $1.20, while another quarter had a cost greater than $4.70. Approximately one-third of the facility costs per participant day were in-kind contributions. When in-kind costs are excluded, the median facility costs are $1.80 across all sites. Auspice Model I centers had a median cost per participant day almost twice that of Auspice Model II centers ($5.20 versus $2.60). As the square footage per participant did not differ significantly between the two auspice models, it is likely that the difference in cost reflects a difference in cost per square foot.

FOOD COSTS

Food costs were the fourth-largest category of expenditures. These costs, incurred in providing meals and snacks, include food items, consumables, labor, and associated nonlabor costs. Among the sample centers, 38.1 percent prepared meals on site, 39.1 percent bought meals from a vendor, and 22.8 percent prepared some and purchased the rest.

The median food cost was $2.40 per participant day, although for one-fourth of the centers the cost per participant day was less than $0.80 and for another one-fourth more than $2.80. Differences in number and kinds of meals served among centers partially account for this wide discrepancy. For example, some centers offered breakfast and/or dinner in addition to a noon meal, while others offered the noon meal only. As with facility costs, a large proportion of the food costs—almost one-half—were in kind.

Median food costs per participant day, like median costs for labor and facilities, were significantly higher for Auspice Model I than for Auspice Model II centers. This difference was probably because Model I Centers were more likely to offer additional meal services.

OTHER COSTS

The remaining categories shown in Table 5.6 are administrative and allo-cated costs. Administrative costs include general administrative supplies; printing and copying; postage; and legal, accounting, and auditing ser-vices, as well as labor costs associated with fiscal managers, bookkeepers, secretaries, or other office personnel. Administrative costs added a median of $1 per participant day.

Allocated costs are those costs that are not incurred directly by the day care operations, but instead are overhead expenses allocated to the center by its parent organization, for example, management-related expenses. The median allocated cost was $1.00, but for those sites that reported some allocated costs, the median allocated cost per participant day was $3.22.

An Examination of Capacity
Adjusted Costs per Participant Day

A major problem with cost per participant day is that it fails to correct for inefficiencies associated with volume. Efficiency is a major concern in de-termining the unit cost of adult day care because so many of the costs asso-ciated with these centers are fixed. Fixed costs do not vary in total with volume, but decline exponentially on a per unit basis as volume increases; thus, cost per participant day may be high, not because the numerator (costs) is high, but because the denominator (participants days) is low. Such a situation occurs when centers provide fewer participant days of service than they have the capacity to provide.

In addition to being asked how many participants the center was li-censed to serve, each center director was asked: "In your opinion, what is the total number of participants able to be served in the present location with current staffing levels?" Responses to this question (reported capacity) from the 22 responding centers (for which complete fiscal data were also available) and their reported average daily census were used to build an index of the percentage of service capacity at which the center was operating.

Using this index, annual participant days at each site were adjusted to equal 100 percent of the reported capacity. Similarly, variable costs for food and transportation were adjusted to reflect volume differences. The variable food cost per participant day was calculated by dividing relevant annual food cost (raw food, consumables, and contracted expenses) by annual participant days. Likewise, the variable transportation cost was calculated by dividing relevant annual transportation costs (gas, maintenance, and contracted transportation expenses) by annual participant days. Remaining costs were assumed to be fixed, and thus not expected to increase with an increase in participant days.

Centers were operating at a median percent capacity of 80 percent with Auspice Model I centers operating at a median of 67 percent and Auspice Model II centers operating at a median of 80 percent of capacity. Before adjustment, the median total cost per participant day was $30.80 for the responding centers. When adjusted to full capacity, however, this cost fell to $23.50, a drop of 20 percent. Before adjustment, Auspice Model I and Auspice Model II sites had a median cost per participant day of $26.40 and $32.00, respectively. After adjustment, Auspice Model I sites dropped 29 percent to $20.70, and Auspice Model II sites dropped 18 percent to $24.60 per participant day.

Even if excess demand existed (as measured by the presence of a waiting list), the centers were not usually operating at full capacity. In his report on adult day care in Massachusetts, Palmer (1983) found a similar phenomenon. He attributed extra capacity to variable absenteeism; that is, staffing was based on capacity even though on many occasions not all participants showed up. This also may be the case among sample centers in this survey.

Thus, two rival hypotheses exist: (1) day care centers are working at full capacity, and any slack results from reserving space for variable absenteeism; or (2) day care centers are operating below capacity because of inefficiencies. Data to test these hypotheses are beyond the scope of this study. However, to the extent the latter hypothesis is true, it is important to know the effects of more efficient operations on cost per participant day. Thus a model was developed to illustrate the economies of scale that might be reached at various levels of capacity utilization. The model is based on assumptions that closely mirror the data found at the 22 participating sites that supplied capacity information. With this model, we found cost per participant day decreased, from $44.35 when operations were at 50 percent of capacity to $23.48 when average daily census rose to full capacity (Figure 5.1).

Note that under the assumptions made here, the average dollar savings to be gained with each unit of increase in average daily census decreases at a declining rate as utilization increases. Thus, the lower the current utilization of operating capacity to begin with, the greater the potential savings to be gained in unit costs for equal gains in utilization. For instance, as average daily census changes from 13 to 14 persons, average cost decreases from $44.35 to $41.37 or $2.98. However, as average daily census changes from 25 to 26, average cost decreases from $24.32 to $23.48, or only $0.83. The cost behavior characteristics shown here are typical of social service and health service centers, each of which tends to have a high proportion of fixed costs.

Because most per diem fees are based on an average cost estimate, one way in which adult day care centers with excess capacity can maximize their net income is by instituting efficiencies based on increased utilization. Whereas reimbursement is based on average cost, each unit of volume increases cost at a lower rate—marginal cost. Thus, if reimbursement per participant day is greater than marginal cost, a profit will be made on each unit of increase in participant days. Exactly how much will depend on the exact amount paid by the reimbursement agency.

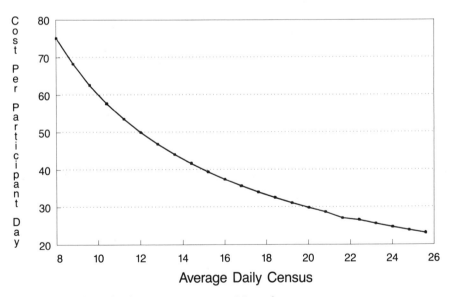

Figure 5.1. Effects of utilization on cost per participant day.

Conclusions

The findings presented here are intended to update current knowledge of the funding and costs of adult day care in the United States. The three sets of findings included: (1) revenues, expenses, and profits; (2) unit revenues and costs; and (3) the possible effects of capacity adjustments. The aggregate analyses provide an overview of the industry as a whole.

Using median data, a profile of a typical site can be constructed as having revenues of approximately $140,000 and expenses that are slightly higher. Most of the revenues come from federal sources, with Medicaid being the largest single source. Auspice Model I centers, many of which are associated with nursing homes and have religious affiliations, are considerably more reliant on nongovernmental funding than are Model II centers, of which a higher proportion are Medicaid certified.

Adult day care is a labor-intensive industry, with labor accounting for more than 50 percent of the costs. Labor, transportation, facility, and food costs together account for the bulk of the industry's expenses. Labor costs constitute a higher proportion of total costs for Model I sites than for Model II sites, perhaps reflecting the more intense services provided to a population that is frailer and more physically dependent.

Over all sites, about 10 percent of expenses were in kind, although in general Model I sites reported only a negligible amount of in-kind expenses. Finally, although across all sites there was a slightly negative median bottom line, the Model I sites were operating with a product margin of 6 percent.

Most centers operate in affiliation with a larger organization, often using what would have been unused space, idle equipment, and underutilized staff. Additional costs to the parent organization associated with running the center therefore are marginal.

The second set of findings focused on the cost per participant day of adult day care centers. The median cost was $29.50, with little difference found between Auspice Model I and Auspice Model II centers.

Although we anticipated finding significant cost differences between the two auspice models, no difference in total cost per participant day was found. Significant differences were found, however, between the cost structure of the two models. This may reflect prevailing reimbursement practices for day that have the effect of capping total revenues, regardless of provider costs. The effect of this cap is that centers with high costs in one cost center, such as physical space in nursing homes or rehabilitation hospitals, must adjust their direct spending on other centers to remain under the revenue "ceiling."

It is interesting to compare the $29.50 median costs per participant day found here to Weissert's 1975 figure of $21.32 (Weissert, 1975). According to these figures, median costs have risen only 40 percent in 11 years, compared to general inflation of 100 percent. The randomness of the 1975 sample may explain some of the differences, but another reason for the minimal increase in the cost of day care may be that many centers are paid on a flat rate basis by many of their funding sources, with no consideration for either costs incurred or inflation. Additional support for this hypothesis is provided by the substantially higher costs found among centers paid by an historical cost reimbursement method (Weissert et al., 1980). This suggests that while day care centers find it difficult to operate without net losses under their current reimbursement system, these systems appear to be effective at holding down costs.

Remembering that the cost per participant day reflects an average of six hours of care per day, or an average hourly cost of approximately $5, adult day care seems to be a bargain. Unfortunately, data collected in this study do not allow us to examine the possible effects of this relative cutback in funds on the centers or their participants.

The final section focused on developing a model to show potential unit cost savings related to increases in utilization of capacity. Two points should be stressed from the information presented in that section: (1) to the extent that adult day care centers are operating below capacity, their per participant day costs may be unnecessarily high; and (2) to the extent that an adult day care center's reimbursable cost is above its marginal cost, each additional participant day represents revenue in excess of expenses.

One important concern with increased efficiency, however, may be reduced satisfaction. Given the findings in the satisfaction chapter there may be trade-offs involved between operating at maximum capacity and achieving highest levels of satisfaction with the center's milieu.

Finally, a note of caution is warranted with respect to cost findings. The factors noted in the methodology section, particularly response rate and self-reported, unaudited data, suggest that care should be exercised in applying these findings beyond the sites included in this analysis.

SIX

CONCLUSIONS

THE NUMBER of adult day care centers has increased during the past decade, paralleling both the secular growth of the dependent elderly population who need supportive services and improved funding prospects under the Medicaid home- and community-based care act of 1981 (U.S. Social Security Act Title XIX, Medicaid, Section 1915c). Political support for day care is also strong, manifested in the willingness of leading members of the U.S. Congress to introduce legislation which, if adopted, would greatly expand public subsidy for day care use by dependent elderly and non-elderly indivdiuals (U.S. Congress, 1988). One of this study's goals was to describe this developing care modality after a decade of growth. (Another goal was to develop microcomputer software to improve center planning and program design—See Appendix.)

Models of Day Care

The National Institute of Adult Day Care uses an appropriately broad definition to describe adult day care (Von Behren, 1986), but this study showed that day care is a heterogeneous concept that can be better understood if the centers are categorized into three distinctive models of care. Who uses a center appears to be influenced by the type of agency with which the center is affiliated.

The following three models appear useful to describe available adult day care.

Auspice Model I centers were defined as affiliated with a nursing home or rehabilitation hospital. They typically provide services to a physically dependent, older, white population, most of whom do not suffer a mental disorder. Nursing, therapies, therapeutic diets, and other health and social services are provided by a complement of staff approaching one staff member for every two participants. Transportation to and from other services, especially health care services, is often available. Revenues come heavily from philanthropic and self-pay sources rather than governmental sources.

Auspice Model II centers were defined as those affilliated with a general hospital or a social services or housing agency. They serve a predominately unmarried and female population, frequently of a racial minority; most are under 85 and are typically not dependent or only minimally dependent in activities of daily living, but more than 40 percent may be suffering a mental disorder. Services include case management, nutrition education, professional counseling, transportation to and from the center, and frequently health assessment. Revenues come heavily from governmental sources, particularly Medicaid.

Special Purpose centers, each serve a single type of clientele such as the blind, the mentally ill, or veterans. Although averages were presented as a point of reference for these programs, their within-group variability makes such summary statistics less meaningful than those for Models I and II.

The profile of a typical day care participant is a 78-year-old, unmarried, white female who does not live alone and is functionally dependent. Participants of Auspice Model I centers, the most physically dependent of the three groups, in general manifested more of the characteristics associated with nursing home institutionalization than elderly participants of either of the other two models. However, day care participants collectively, and in each of the three models, differed sharply from typical nursing home residents.

Printed program materials and center directors' questionnaire responses nonetheless indicated that one of the many purposes of day care centers was to delay or prevent institutionalization. Directors also emphasized social interaction and recreation, rehabilitative training/skill building, or health monitoring and maintenance. In the view of the study team, what centers most often do—at least at a minimum—is offer individuals a place to go during the day where social interaction, exercise, and a hot noontime meal are available, and where nursing observation and supervision are provided.

Utilization

The average daily census at centers varied from under 6 to over 40, averaging just under 20 participants a day. In general, Model II centers had the largest daily census of the three models. Elderly participants attended for an average of almost three and one-half days per week and for just under six hours per day. Multivariate analysis of participant frequency of participation data suggests that attendance is influenced by auspice model, participant characteristics, and community variables.

In most instances, those attending centers affiliated with nursing homes and rehabilitation hospitals attended day care less frequently than participants of centers affiliated with other types of agencies.

Of particular interest is the differential effect of the interaction between center type and individual characteristics on frequency of attendance. A single characteristic may increase or reduce the frequency of attendance, depending on the auspices of the center that a participant with that characteristic attends. For example, a participant with impaired mobility has an increased chance of full-time attendance if he or she attends an Auspice Model I center, while the same person has a reduced probability of full-time attendance if he or she attends an Auspice Model II center.

Frequency of participation among Medicaid participants appeared to be sensitive to participant needs; for example, more dependent participants had an increased likelihood of full-time attendance compared to less dependent participants. These findings support the notion that Medicaid is a prudent buyer of adult day care services.

Transportation, the single center service introduced in the model, did not appear to influence frequency of participation, although access to transportation has previously been found to have a substantial impact on use or nonuse of day care services.

Finally, county characteristics, such as competition among day care providers, and center characteristics, such as the efficiency of service delivery (capacity of maximal operations achieved), did appear to influence frequency of participation. To fully understand these county and center effects, further research is needed to test causal relationships based on detailed data on service costs, supply, and competition.

Satisfaction

The success of a day care center ultimately may rest on factors that influence satisfaction and continued utilization. Although most of the participants were satisfied with the overall program, and with specific aspects of the program, slightly less than a quarter of the sample was completely satisfied with all aspects of day care, leading one to believe that satisfaction with one aspect counterbalances dissatisfaction with another.

Factor analysis was used to identify three types of satisfaction: structural dimensions, intrinsic quality, and center milieu. The three types of satisfaction measured different aspects of day care, and it is not surprising that the program and participant characteristics found to correlate with each were also different.

Findings indicate that whites and older participants tended to be the most satisfied with the first factor—structural conditions of the center. However, those who lived alone or who had symptoms, signs, or ill-defined conditions were less satisfied with the structural conditions of day care, and appeared to be more sensitive to such issues as transportation, program hours, quality of food, and center temperature.

Participants with symptoms, signs, or ill-defined conditions also appear to be the most difficult to satisfy intrinsically. There is no clear reason why they do not feel well, and their response to the center is more negative than other types of participants.

Intrinsic satisfaction also is related to the number of staff available. The greater the staff (more than one therapist and nurse), the more satisfied were the participants with the attention they received and with the program itself. In addition to staff size, the participants' general level of life satisfaction was found to positively correlate with intrinsic satisfaction with the center.

In terms of the last component of satisfaction analyzed, that of center milieu, those participants likely to be less satisfied with the noise level and crowdedness were those who had endocrine disorders, paid privately, and used centers where there were more staff. The effect of average daily attendance was also negatively related to dissatisfaction with the center's milieu.

This finding illustrates an interesting dilemma for day care centers and directors. The participant's intrinsic satisfaction increases with more staff, for they like the attention they can receive for their needs; however, they do not like the accompanying noise and more crowded feeling.

In addition to high levels of participant satisfaction, at-home caregivers also reported high levels of satisfaction with day care. The high levels of satisfaction found among participants and caregivers supports the idea that day care appears to be meeting the needs of its clientele, particularly caregivers who are trying to balance family commitments and their own work.

Regulation

More than half of the centers reported holding at least one license, and more than half were certified. In general, centers were licensed as either adult day health programs or social or nonspecific adult day care centers, and the most common licensing agency was the state health department. Although certification can be required for a number of types of funding, the most common funding source was Medicaid, and the state Medicaid office was the most frequent certifying agency.

Consistent with these perceptions, regulated centers differed from their unregulated counterparts in the following ways:

- Certified centers were more likely to employ more and more skilled staff per participant;
- Both certified and licensed centers were more likely to offer various services;
- Regulated centers were more likely to be housed in facilities that met 504 standards and were used exclusively for day care;
- Regulated centers served participants who attended more frequently and in larger numbers;
- Regulated centers served participants who were more likely to be publicly subsidized, of racial minorities, unmarried, and younger than those served in unregulated centers.

In the opinion of center directors, meeting regulatory standards frequently required changes in many or most of the components of established centers' operations, and often affected program costs. Typically, these changes were viewed as necessary by the directors. One of the most common and costly changes required for regulatory compliance was in staffing. Licensure and certification standards addressed both staff-to-participant ratios and skill mix.

Our findings suggest that, although varying from state to state, both licensure and certification affect many aspects of center operations, and that making the necessary changes for compliance probably involves some costs. However, it appears that centers that comply and acquire licensure or certification may be rewarded with a larger census, probably because publicly subsidized participants are more likely to attend licensed and certified centers.

Financing

Efforts to collect detailed financial data revealed that the financial reporting/accounting procedures of the adult day care industry are underdeveloped. Nonetheless, the data available show a typical center had revenues of approximately $140,000 per year and expenses that were slightly higher. Most revenues came from federal sources, with Medicaid being the largest single source. Model I programs, many of which were associated with nursing homes and had religious affiliations, were considerably more reliant on nongovernmental funding than were Model II programs.

The median total cost per participant day was $29.50, and although the range was quite great, half the sites incurred a daily cost between $23.40 and $36.10. More than half the expenses were attributable to labor costs. Labor costs at Model I sites tended to constitute a higher proportion of total costs than for Model II sites, perhaps reflecting the more intense services provided to a population that was frailer and more physically dependent.

Although component cost per participant day did differ between the two Auspice Models, the total cost per participant day did not differ. This perhaps reflects prevailing reimbursement practices for care that have the effect of capping total revenues, regardless of costs.

Keeping in mind that the cost per participant day reflects an average of six hours of care per day, or an average hourly cost of approximately $5, adult day care currently seems to be a bargain. This is especially true if one considers that the cost of day care has risen only 40 percent since 1975, compared to general inflation of approximately 100 percent for the same time period. Additionally, to the extent that centers are operating below capacity, potential to lower the cost per day may exist.

Conclusions

Adult day care has, for more than 10 years, maintained a place for itself in this country as one option in the continuum of care for the chronically ill and disabled. Appropriately, as the heterogeneity of the population it serves demands, day care is varied and changing.

Results of this national survey showed that the day care market is beginning to be differentiated further as it matures—expanding to three principal types of centers. The most recent of these to develop is the most specialized, and is targeted to individuals manifesting homogeneous needs. Further differentiation of the market might be expected as the growing chronically ill population becomes large enough to support more specialized centers.

Costs of day care have remained low, but possibly could be reduced even further if increased demand enhanced their ability to operate closer to capacity. Increased demand is likely if legislation recently introduced in Congress to expand Medicare coverage to include adult day care is passed.

But one important trade-off of increasing demand, and thus efficiency, may be reduced satisfaction. Conclusions from the satisfaction analysis show that center milieu is one area that already is amenable to improvement, and increasing operations to capacity would likely increase the noise level and crowdedness of the center.

The computer software we have available as one product of our study may help day care centers improve their efficiency by being better able to project effects of various organizational choices on costs, revenues, profitability, and financial viability. (See the Appendix for a detailed description of DayCare, the computer software.)

Finally, this national study offered several indications that day care will continue to play a role, and one that is increasingly important, in the long-term care continuum. Day care appears well positioned to help meet the needs of its clients as well as the growing demand for programs to support the family caregiver. It appears flexible enough to respond to market changes, and has such a favorable cost structure that it is reasonable to assume that it will continue to flourish and change as the needs of its client populations change.

DayCare: A Computer-Assisted System for Planning Adult Day Care Centers

To this point we have concentrated on describing the day care industry. In this appendix, the focus shifts to how to change it. In many respects, the preceding analyses were conducted as background to the main purpose of the study, which was to develop a decision-support software program that would help day care center operators develop more efficient day care centers. Using the conceptual model of day care presented in Chapter 1 as a framework, data from the national survey were incorporated into a software package.

This software is designed to help current or potential operators of day care centers consider the consequences for program costs of each organizational decision which must be made—everything from the choice of auspice to expected daily census, staffing, or services to be provided. Choices about whether or not to provide services directly or under contract are also considered. Decision options are presented to the software user for each organizational choice that must be made. In each case, averages and ranges from the survey data, tailored to the program being designed, are presented for use as guidelines.

Using the software, one can anticipate the effects of a change in average daily census, the tasks which are to be performed by a staff member, or other changes. The effects of these changes on costs, their offsetting effects on revenues, and in turn the consequences for the center's net profitability are recalculated automatically by the software.

The expectation is that the software will be used to consider the consequences of an organizational choice, to conduct a sensitivity analysis of the effects of alternative choices, and, ultimately, to make choices that are most likely to maximize the efficiency of the center's program. Of particular value may be the potential for users to avoid unrealistic expectations for census, staff, expenses, scope of services, revenues, or other operational estimates.

The software is available for only a nominal reproduction and shipping charge, is not copyrighted, and is designed for the operator with little or no computer experience.

The Planning System
for Adult Day Care

DayCare is a computer software system designed to assist operators in planning new adult day care centers and in adapting existing centers to changing circumstances. The software was developed with funds from the John A. Hartford Foundation by the Program on Aging in the School of Public Health at The University of North Carolina-Chapel Hill, with assistance from 3C, Inc. of Durham, N.C. Principal designers were Ms. Elise Bolda and Mr. Teiji Kimball, who implemented the vision of the principal investigator, Dr. William Weissert, for this planning tool.

With DayCare, users can anticipate characteristics of the participant population, make staffing choices, estimate costs, and analyze revenues. DayCare takes the user through such major planning issues as whether to hire a full-time registered nurse, whether to contract for transportation or to use facility-owned vehicles, and whether to prepare meals on site or to contract for them. The software shows the effects each decision would have on center operations; thus, choices can be evaluated before they are implemented.

Users can also calculate the effects of changes in daily census and of changes in revenues or costs on planned or established centers. Daycare can present alternatives for adapting to such changes, and users can try out different solutions to problems before altering established policies and practices or instituting new ones.

By assisting users in making informed planning decisions, Daycare systematically asks users critical questions so that they can frame operation of new centers or evaluate existing programs.

Hardware Required

DayCare will operate on any IBM or truly compatible microcomputer that has 640K actual memory available. It is easier to operate on computers with hard disk drives; however, it will run on some double floppy drive systems. Two software disks are used to operate DayCare, a Master disk and a System disk. User-supplied information is automatically saved to a formatted blank disk at the conclusion of each session.

Using the Software

DayCare is a user-friendly, menu-driven system. The program is arranged for flexibility and experimentation. Main menu selections are identified for the four major sections of DayCare: Operations Data, Labor Data, Other Expense Data, and Revenue Data. The main menu sections are further divided into more specific subsections where detailed questions are asked and summaries are provided.

The software has two initial selections for beginning the software, the Default mode or the New View mode. The Default mode, with preset values for all entry choices, serves as a tutorial, providing a trial run through the program. For users interested in a freestanding center (e.g., centers not operating under the auspices of a larger organization), which is not reimbursed by Medicaid, the Default mode can also be used as an actual file and may be modified by the user. DayCare always retains the original Default file and requires users to rename the file before beginning to prevent altering that file's tutorial features.

In the New View mode, the user must enter all values. The New View mode is designed to accommodate centers that are operated independently or in affiliation with other programs, and accommodates centers that do and those that do not receive Medicaid reimbursement.

The following sections review the sequential menu selections and subsections that comprise the DayCare software system design. See Figure A.1 for a diagram of the full system design.

OPERATIONS DATA

The first major section in the software asks the user to begin a file by entering personal information (User Data), and data about a program (Program Data) and its participants (Case Mix Data), either actual or anticipated.

Program Data The software asks the user to classify the day care program as freestanding (independent) or affiliated with one of the following types of organizations: nursing home, rehabilitation facility, senior citizen program, housing authority, social services agency, or general hospital. From this response, DayCare selects which Auspice Model average and range data from the national survey will be presented to the user throughout the software program. If the user selects affiliation with either a nursing home or rehabilitation facility, data presented will be from Auspice Model I programs, which serve more functionally dependent participants. If other affiliations are selected, DayCare will display data from Auspice

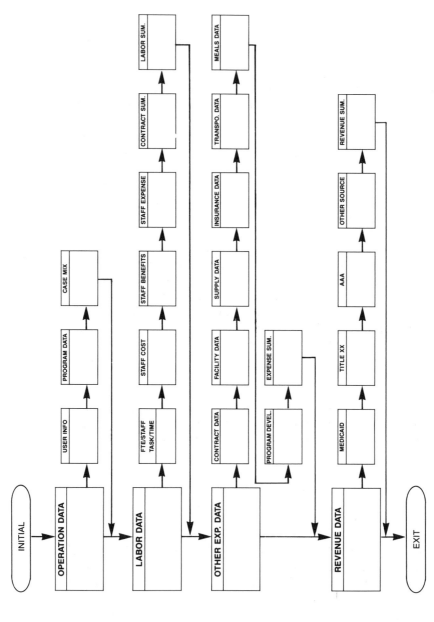

Figure A.1. *DayCare* software system design.

Model II programs, which generally serve less dependent participants. (The Auspice Models are discussed in detail in Chapter 1.)

After deciding affiliation, the user is asked whether Medicaid reimbursement for center services is anticipated. Again, DayCare uses the response to select data to be displayed with individual questions throughout the software. Information displayed depends on whether the center will or will not receive Medicaid reimbursement, because program expenses and revenues are influenced by Medicaid certification requirements.

Users are informed that Medicaid reimbursement is not available in all states and that requirements for Medicaid reimbursement vary by state. Medicaid and State Daycare Association contact lists are presented in the Appendix of the DayCare Users Manual, and users are encouraged to seek specific information about their state.

Within the Program Data section, users are also asked whether they intend to serve participants who are younger than 60 years. Because many centers receive financial support from Area Agencies on Aging through the Older Americans Act, users are informed about federal rules governing eligibility for these funds. Although additional detail about the percent of nonelderly participants is requested in the Area Agency on Aging revenue subsection, users are reminded that revenue from this source is limited to expenses associated with serving only elderly participants.

Once affiliation and Medicaid reimbursement have been decided, DayCare asks for the number of people who will be enrolled in the center; the number of participants expected, on average, to attend each day; the number of days per week the center will be open; and the number of days each year the center will operate. The user is presented with national averages and ranges for each value requested, based on the survey results from centers of similar affiliations and Medicaid reimbursement status.

Program Data information is used throughout the Daycare program and must be entered before other sections are approached. DayCare uses these values in computing, for example, labor needed, meal and transportation costs, space required, revenues, and unit costs per participant day.

Case Mix   The final subsection in Operations Data refers to participants and their levels of dependency. Users are asked to enter average percentages of participants who fall within the following categories: independent in all activities of daily living; dependent in toileting or eating; and dependent in mobility. The software then asks for percentages of participants who live alone and who have a mental disability. For each question, DayCare displays the average and range from the national survey for similar centers, that is, centers of similar affiliation and Medicaid reimbursement status.

Finally, DayCare provides a summary of the user's responses to questions in the Operations Data menu (the affiliation selected; Medicaid reimbursement status; whether nonelderly persons are expected to be served; estimated enrollment and average daily census; annual operating days; and detail on participant characteristics from the case-mix subsection.)

LABOR DATA

Staff/Task/Time   In its staffing section, rather than arbitrary staffing patterns DayCare uses an estimation approach that enables the projection of staffing needs based on participant needs. Users are asked to select potential positions from lists of Administrative, Non-Medical, Therapeutic, and Ancillary professions and paraprofessions. Data on the percentage of programs that employed or contracted for staff in each position are provided.

Users are then asked to estimate time required for the performance of specific tasks displayed in four categories: Management, Facilitative, Direct Participant Care, and Other. Each of these is further subdivided into specific "subtasks." For example, within management, employees could be responsible for some or all of the following: marketing, reporting, budgeting, personnel, fundraising, and billing/payables. Users are asked how many hours per week (if any) will be allocated to the performance of each task listed.

DayCare provides average and range values in units requested by the software: hours per week for Management and Facilitative tasks, or minutes per participant per day for Direct Participant Care tasks. DayCare converts minutes per participant day to hours per week on the basis of the number of participants served daily and days of operation previously entered by the user. Data for time estimates are from a subsample of centers from the national survey in which day care center staff estimated the time spent for tasks listed. Estimates from the national survey include "downtime" within the allocated task times.

For each position selected, the user then assigns responsibility for task performance and the amount of time, if any, that the user feels is appropriate for each position to spend on the task. DayCare subtracts the assigned time from the corresponding position, and maintains a running balance of unassigned time (e.g., total task time allocated minus time already assigned to a position), which is displayed throughout the position task time assignment section.

For both the position and task lists, users are allowed to enter their own position or task description and estimates. DayCare incorporates these "customized" entries throughout the remainder of the program.

– 110 –

Finally, based on user-defined full-time status, Daycare computes how many full-time equivalent people are needed for each selected position. The advantage of this approach is that staff are appropriately estimated based on work to be performed, rather than guessing what would be the most efficient staffing levels.

The remaining subsections of the Labor Data menu use the results of the Staff/Task/Time subsection and report only choices or estimates entered by the user.

Staff Cost The user specifies hourly rates for each position selected. Daycare provides the average hourly rates from the national survey for reference.

Fringe Benefits Employee benefits can be estimated on the basis of a flat rate or by a detailing annual premium expenses. Eligibility for fringe benefits, defined by hours per week worked, is supplied by the user.

Staff Expense Daycare presents the number of full-time equivalents estimated by the user, based on the user defined hours per week for a full-time worker. For this list of full- and part-time staff, the user must decide whether personnel required will be employed directly by the center or under contract and may modify the hourly payment rate to reflect more senior status or experience of individual staff holding the same position.

Contract Labor Summary The Contract Labor Summary provides a list of all contract personnel and computes the annual contract labor costs, and contract labor costs per participant day. If no contracted labor has been identified, the user cannot access the Contract Labor Summary.

Labor Summary Both direct employees and contract labor are reviewed in this subsection. Detail on annual costs for each position, fringe benefit costs (if appropriate), and total labor expense is displayed. In addition, several staff to participant ratios are computed and national values are provided for comparison.

OTHER EXPENSE DATA

In the third major section, the user supplies information on contract costs for meal and transportation services; costs of providing and maintaining the physical facility; expenses for supplies, insurance, and program-provided transportation; on-site meal preparation and raw food costs; and other expenses.

Contract Data The first subsection asks for estimated costs of contracted meals and transportation. The user enters the estimated cost per participant per meal or trip and the percent of participants expected to receive the services. Averages and ranges from the national survey are provided as guidelines.

After all information is entered, DayCare provides summaries of total contract meal and transportation expenses and costs per participant day for each contracted service.

Facility Data In the second subsection in Other Expense Data, the user enters estimated costs for monthly rent or mortgage payments and utilities. As with other sections, Daycare provides the user with national estimates for these expenses based on programs similar to the one being estimated.

If the space housing the center is rented or leased, the user may enter either monthly expenses or cost per square foot and square footage per participant, and DayCare will estimate total area needed and the subsequent monthly and annual expense. If the program owns the space, or is purchasing it through a mortgage, the user is asked to enter monthly payments and information used to compute annual depreciation. Monthly utilities costs, including costs for water, sewer, electricity, heating, air conditioning, and maintenance may be entered separately if they are not included in rental arrangements.

DayCare summarizes the costs for the building and the utilities, and the cost per participant per day for space.

Supply Data The next subsection includes cost estimates for participant activity supplies, therapeutic supplies, and office expenses in separate submenus. DayCare asks the user for the cost per participant per day or total monthly supply expense for each category. Based on user-supplied information, DayCare calculates the total monthly cost or cost per participant per day (whichever is not entered by the user) and annual expense. In the Office Data Menu, monthly telephone expenses are estimated in addition to the costs of cleaning and general office supplies.

The supply summary is comprehensive, including the total annual cost of supplies as well as the cost of supplies per participant day.

Insurance Data In the fourth subsection under Other Expense Data, the user supplies annual premium costs for insurance, including staff liability, general liability, fire and theft, and other. Data displayed by DayCare are limited in this section because of the complexity of insurance coverages. Users are urged to seek local insurance estimates for detailed coverage as there are vast differences in premium prices across states.

Transportation Data In this subsection, the software asks for all expenses the center expects to incur in owning and operating vehicles. Here, the user enters the percentage of program participants who need to be transported.

Next, the user enters the number of vehicles the center uses or plans to use (whether owned or leased), the monthly payment associated with each, annual insurance premium costs, and information for estimating depreciation if appropriate. For vehicles being purchased, DayCare computes a straight line depreciation expense.

DayCare asks for estimates of gasoline price, mileage per day, miles per gallon of gasoline, costs of annual maintenance, annual registration expense, and licensing expense for each vehicle. The transportation summary provides the total annual expense for direct transportation, the cost per trip, and the cost per participant day.

Meals Data This is the subsection in which the user enters the costs of on-site snack and meal preparation. DayCare first asks for percentages of participants who will be served breakfast, lunch, dinner, or snacks. The user then enters the cost for raw food and consumables (paper goods, plates, cups, etc.) per meal and other equipment expenses. The software provides national averages and computes total annual expenses for both raw foods and consumables. DayCare then summarizes total annual meal expenses and the cost per participant per day. DayCare also provides a cost-per-lunch estimate to enable the user to compare the expense of on-site meal preparation with that of contracted meal services.

To limit meals served or transportation provided to the logical 100 percent of participants, the contract and direct service subsections for meals and transportation are linked within DayCare. Therefore, to compare on-site meal preparation or direct transportation services with contracted meal or transportation expenses, users must either use separate DayCare files or enter less than 51 percent served in each section (Contract Data or Transportation/Meal Data).

Program Development In this subsection, the user enters projected start-up costs, including legal fees, accounting expenses, first-year equipment payments, other equipment depreciation costs, and overhead expenses.

Expense Summary The final subsection of the Other Expense menu provides the line-item annual expenses in dollars and as a percent of the total annual expense, including salaries, benefits, contracted labor, contracted services, facilities and utilities, supplies, telephone, insurances, vehicle expenses, vehicle depreciation, gas, licenses, vehicle maintenance, raw food, consumables, legal fees, accounting, and other costs. The format of the expense summary is an annual projected budget, and it includes estimated costs per participant per day.

The Expense Summary is a critical part of DayCare because it allows operators to evaluate their major cost centers (labor, meals, transportation, and facility) and compare the percentages of their expenses in each category with the average and range values from the national survey. Such comparison will provide a basis for determining whether individual estimates are high or low in relation to those we found during the survey.

REVENUE DATA

In the final section, the user enters revenue estimates. This section includes subsections for revenues from Medicaid, Social Services Block Grants (Title XX), Area Agencies on Aging (Older Americans Act), and other sources such as private payment, United Way, and community contributions.

Medicaid   Information concerning Medicaid can be entered only if the user has indicated, in the Operations Data section, that the center is eligible to receive Medicaid reimbursements. If the center expects Medicaid reimbursement, the user enters the estimated percentage of participants eligible for reimbursement and the hourly or daily rate of reimbursement. Users are also offered the option of estimating supplemental payments for therapies or transportation if they are not included in the hourly or daily reimbursement rate. An optional feature asks users what cost centers are allowed in determining the Medicaid reimbursement rate if reimbursement is cost based. Information about state Medicaid policies is helpful to users in completing this section, although, as in other sections, national survey data are displayed.

When all pertinent information has been entered, DayCare supplies a summary of totals for annual revenue from base (hourly, per diem or cost based reimbursement) and supplemental payments, and computes total Medicaid revenue, the total per diem reimbursement rate (in dollars per person per day) for eligible participants, and the percent of total expenses covered by the estimated Medicaid reimbursement.

Title XX   In the Title XX subsection, as with Medicaid, the user enters an estimate of the number of participants eligible for Social Services Block Grants/Title XX funds and the daily or monthly rates of reimbursement. Users have the option of including supplemental meals or transportation payment information. If Social Service Block Grant funds are not based on per diem or per month reimbursement schedules, the user has the option to estimate cost-based reimbursement revenue.

The summary of Title XX funds provides total revenue, per diem reimbursement per eligible participant, and the percentage of total annual expenses covered by the estimated Title XX revenue.

Area Agency on Aging In the third subsection of the Revenue menu, the percentage of participants eligible for Area Agency on Aging (AAA) funding under the Older Americans Act (OAA) is entered. The user may enter total dollar value applied to meal or transportation expenses or the percent of actual costs covered. The user also specifies whether this support is paid in cash or as donated (in-kind) contributions. The amount of non-specific grant funds the center expects to receive and value of Senior Community Service Labor are also options for user entry. The summary provides the total annual revenue from Older Americans Act funds and the estimated revenue, both per participant per day and as a percent of total expenses.

Other Sources In this subsection the user estimates revenues from such sources as United Way, private payments, and other contributions and donations. Private payments are estimated in a manner similar to that used in the Medicaid and Social Service Block Grant sections. The user estimates percent of participants making payment and the average per diem payment. The summary of Other Sources of revenue includes annual revenue from each source, revenue per participant day, and Other Source revenues as a percent of total expenses.

Revenue Summary The final subsection shows what percentage of all revenues can be expected from each source which has been entered. Day-Care also displays the national average and range values so that operators can view their revenue mix (the proportion of total revenue by source). In addition, DayCare provides a summary of total projected annual expenses and revenues for the day care center and computes the "bottom line" by subtracting expenses from revenues. This information allows operators to anticipate the center's success or failure in terms of dollars and cents. Finally, an advice screen provides suggestions for reducing expenses and increasing revenues, if expenses exceed revenues.

Summary

DayCare was designed to assist operators in planning new adult day care centers and in continuing efficient operations of established centers in the face of changing circumstances. Averages and norms based on data from the national survey are displayed for easy reference throughout the software. The software is user friendly and flexible. Users can choose one of two modes, Default or New View. The Default mode incorporates preset values and can be used as a preliminary tutorial.

The four major sections of DayCare (Operations Data, Labor Data, Other Expense Data, and Revenue Data) are sequential, but the user can easily return to previous menus to make changes and corrections. Day-Care saves information automatically, and summaries can be printed on request. The Revenue Summary, a comprehensive assessment of annual expenses and revenues, is the basis for the final screen, which provides advice concerning changes the center can make to improve its financial outlook.

DayCare has several features designed for user ease:

- It is a sequential program; the user begins in Operations Data and ends in Revenue Data;
- It is flexible; the user can access different data sections in any order, although for initial entry it is recommended that information be entered in sequence to avoid omitting important estimates;
- The user may, for menu or subsection selection, either move the highlighted cursor to the item choice or type the letter appearing in front of the menu or subsection desired;
- Users may back up to previous sections to make corrections or change values entered;
- Each user input screen contains an instruction/information section;
- Questions to users include national average and range responses from similar programs;
- Each screen contains bottom-line prompts to remind the user what they are asked to do;
- Files are named by the users at the beginning of each session;
- Files are automatically stored;
- Previously established files can be recalled and modified at the users' discretion;
- User-provided information has been restricted to values within predefined ranges to limit errors in data entry and to ensure that no inappropriately large or small values are used;
- Users are repeatedly reminded that their common sense and experience cannot be replaced by the computer software package.

DayCare is available from the Johns Hopkins University Press.

Table A.1
Characteristics of Nonelderly Adult Day Care Participants

	Average age	Female	White	Married	Living alone	Mental disorder[a]	ADL dependencies		IADL dependencies		Prior inpatient use		
							None[b]	Average number	None[c]	Average number	Nursing home (ever)	Mental hospital (ever)	Hospital (within 12 months)
Overall	55.4	45.7%	66.4%	31.4%	17.9%	43.2%	23.2%	2.7	26.0%	1.7	14.3%	11.2%	44.9%
Auspice Model I	54.8	44.2	59.3	57.3+	15.1	17.2	9.0	3.5	41.2	0.8	38.8*	6.5	55.9
Auspice Model II	55.5	50.5	65.1	15.9+	20.6	61.9*	30.8	2.2	22.9	1.9	3.5	12.5	48.8
Special Purpose	56.3	32.7	82.9	37.2	14.2	29.8	27.0	2.5	7.8	2.5*	4.3	15.6	13.0

Note: Includes only individuals under the age of 65; $n = 104$.
[a]Includes ICD-9 codes 290–319.
[b]Person receives no human assistance with bathing, dressing, toileting, transferring, continence, or eating.
[c]Person receives no human assistance with mobility, meal preparation, money management, shopping, or administering medications.
*, Indicates that value is significantly ($p < .05$) different from other two day care model values.
+, Indicates that pairwise difference is significant ($p < .05$).

REFERENCES

Aldrich, J. H., & F. D. Nelson. 1986. *Linear Probability, Logit, and Probit Models*. Quantitative Applications in the Social Sciences Series. Beverly Hills, Calif.: Sage Publications.

Aday, L. A., & R. M. Andersen. 1974. "A Framework for the Study of Access to Medical Care." *Health Services Research* 9:208–20.

Benjamin, A. E. 1986. "Determinants of State Variations in Home Health Utilization and Expenditures Under Medicare." *Medical Care* 24:535–47.

Birnbaum, J. 1981. "Fiscal Management and Reimbursement." In *The Day Hospital: Organization and Management,* ed. C. M. Hamill, 91–98. New York: Springer.

Branch, L. G., & A. M. Jette. 1982. "A Prospective Study of Long-term Care Institutionalization among the Aged." *American Journal of Public Health* 72:1373–79.

Branch, L. G., T. T. Wetle, P. A. Scherr, N. R. Cook, D. A. Evans, L. E. Hebert, E. N. Masland, M. E. Keough, & J. O. Taylor. 1988. "A Prospective Study of Incident Comprehensive Medical Home Care Use among the Elderly." *American Journal of Public Health* 78:255–59.

Brock, A. M., & P. O'Sullivan. 1985. "A Study to Determine What Variables Predict Institutionalization of Elderly People." *Journal of Advanced Nursing* 10:533–37.

Cafferata, G. L. 1987. "Marital Status, Living Arrangements, and the Use of Health Services by Elderly Persons." *Journal of Gerontology* 42:613–18.

Cohen, M. A., E. J. Tell, & S. S. Wallack. 1986. "Client-Related Risk Factors of Nursing Home Entry Among Elderly Adults." *Journal of Gerontology* 41: 785–92.

Conrad, K. J., Hughes, S. C., Campione, P. F., & P. S. Goldberg. 1987. Shedding New Light on Adult Day Care. *Perspective on Aging* 16:18–21.

Coulton, C., & A. K. Frost. 1982. "Use of Social and Health Services by the Elderly." *Journal of Health and Social Behavior* 23:330–39.

Day, P., & R. Klein. 1987. "The Regulation of Nursing Homes: A Comparative Perspective." *Milbank Memorial Fund Quarterly* 65(3):303–47.

Department of Health and Human Services. 1980. *Directory of Adult Day Care Centers.* Health Standards and Quality Bureau: Baltimore, Md.

DiMatteo, M. R., & R. Hays. 1980. "The Significance of Patients' Perceptions of Physician Conduct." *Journal of Community Health* 6:18.

Evashwick, C., G. Rowe, P. Diehr, & L. Branch. 1984. "Factors Explaining the Use of Health Care Services by the Elderly." *Health Services Research* 19: 357–82.

Gray, L. C. 1980. "Consumer Satisfaction with Physician Provided Services: A Panel Study." *Social Science Medicine* 14A:65.

Greenley, J. R., & R. A. Schoenherr. 1981. "Organization Effects on Client Satisfaction with Humaneness of Service." *Journal of Health and Social Behavior* 22:2–18.

Grimaldi, P. L. 1984. "How Major Regulations Serve to Ensure Quality Care in Nursing Homes." *Health Care Financial Management*, September:50–66.

Hannan, E. L., & J. F. O'Donnell. 1984. "Adult Day Care Services in New York State: A Comparison with Other Long-term Care Providers." *Inquiry* 21: 75–83.

Harder, W. P., J. C. Gornick, & M. R. Burt. 1986. "Adult Day Care: Substitute or Supplement?" *Milbank Memorial Fund Quarterly* 64(3):414–41.

Hawes, C., R. H. Kane, L. L. Powers, & J. R. Reinhardy. 1988. "The Case for a Continuum of Long-term Care Services: Lessons from the Community-Based Care Demonstrations." Public Policy Institute of the American Association of Retired Persons, Washington, D.C.

Hulka, B. S., & J. R. Wheat. 1985. "Patterns of Utilization: The Patient Perspective." *Medical Care* 23:438–59.

Hulka, B. S., L. L. Kupper, M. B. Daly, J. C. Cassel, & F. Schoen. 1975. "Correlates of Satisfaction and Dissatisfaction with Medical Care: A Community Perspective." *Medical Care* 13(8):648–58.

Kane, R. A., & R. L. Kane. 1981. *Assessing the Elderly: A Practical Guide to Measurement.* Lexington, Ky.: Lexington Books.

Krout, J. 1983. "Correlates of Senior Center Utilization." *Research on Aging* 5:339–52.

Kurland, C. H. 1982. "The Medical Day Care Program in New Jersey." *Home Health Care Services Quarterly* 3(2):45–61.

Lawton, M. P. and L. Nahemow. 1979. "Social Areas and the Well-being of Tenants in Housing for the Elderly." *Multivariate Behavioral Research* 14: 463–84.

Link, C., S. Long and R. Settle. 1980. "Cost-sharing, Supplementary Insurance, and Health Services Utilization Among the Medicare Elderly." *Health Care Financing Review* 2:25–31.

Linn, M. W., B. S. Linn, & S. R. Stein. 1982. "Satisfaction with Ambulatory Care and Compliance in Older Patients." *Medical Care* 20:606–14.

Lloyd, S., and N. T. Greenspan. 1985. "Nursing Homes, Home Health Services, and Adult Day Care." In *Long-term Care: Perspectives from Research and Demonstrations,* ed. R. J. Vogel & H. C. Palmer, 133–66. Rockville, Md.: Aspen Systems Corporation.

Luft, H. S. 1985. "Competition and Regulation." *Medical Care* 23:383–400.

Mace, N. L., & P. V. Rabins. 1984. *Day Care for Demented Adults.* Washington, D.C.: National Institute for Adult Day Care of the National Council on Aging, Inc.

Mahler, J. 1981. "Barriers to Coordinating Health Services Regulatory Programs." *Journal of Health Politics, Policy and Law* 6:528–41.

Manning, W. G., J. P. Newhouse, N. Duan, E. B. Keeler, A. Leibowitz, & M. S.

Marquis. 1987. "Health Insurance and the Demand for Medical Care: Evidence from a Randomized Experiment." *American Economic Review* 77:251–77.

Marquis, M. S., A. R. Davies, & J. E. Ware. 1983. "Patient Satisfaction and Change in Medical Care Provider: A Longitudinal Study." *Medical Care* 21(8):821–29.

McCoy, J. L., & B. E. Edwards. 1981. "Contextual and Demographic Antecedents of Institutionalization among Aged Welfare Recipients." *Medical Care* 19:907–21.

Moos, R., & S. Lemke. 1984. *The Multiphasic Environmental Assessment Procedure.* Stanford, Calif.: Social Ecology Laboratory, Stanford University School of Medicine.

Mutran, E., & K. F. Ferraro. 1988. "Medical Need and Use of Services among Older Men and Women." *Journal of Gerontology: Social Sciences* 43:S162–71.

National Center for Health Statistics. 1979. Data from the National Health Survey: The National Nursing Home Survey; *Vital and Health Statistics* Ser. 13, No. 43. DHEW Publication No. (PHS) 79-1794.

Novick, L. J. 1973. "Day Care Meets Geriatric Needs." *Journal of American Hospital Association* November:47–50.

Palmer, H. C. 1983. "Adult Day Care." In *Long-Term Care: Perspectives from Research and Demonstration,* ed. R. J. Vogel and H. C. Palmer, 415–36. Rockville, Md.: Aspen Systems Corporation.

Pegels, C. 1980. "Regulations and Controls for Nursing Homes." In *Health Care and Elderly,* 111–15. Rockville, Md.: Aspen Systems Corporation.

Pfeiffer, E. 1975. "A Short Portable Mental Status Questionnaire for the Assessment of Organic Brain Deficit in Elderly Patients." *Journal of American Geriatric Society* 23:433–41.

Pope, C. R. 1978. "Consumer Satisfaction in a Health Maintenance Organization." *Journal of Health and Social Behavior* 19:291–303.

Rathbone-McCuan, E. 1976. "Geriatric Day Care: A Family Perspective." *Gerontologist* 16(6):517–21.

Romm, F. J., & B. S. Hulka. 1979. "Care Process and Patient Outcomes in Diabetes Mellitus." *Medical Care* 17:748.

Roos, N., & E. Shapiro. 1981. "The Manitoba Longitudinal Study on Aging: Preliminary Findings on Health Care Utilization by the Elderly." *Medical Care* 19:644–57.

Ruchlin, H. 1977. "A New Strategy for Regulating Long-term Care Facilities." *Journal of Health Politics, Policy and Law* 2:190–211.

Ruchlin, H. 1979. "An Analysis of Regulatory Issues and Options." In *Long Term Care,* ed. V. LaPorte and J. Rubin, 81–125. New York: Praeger.

Sands, D., & B. S. Suzuki. 1983. "Adult Day Care for Alzheimer's Patients and Their Families." *Gerontologist* 23(1):21–23.

Scanlon, W. J. 1980. "A Theory of the Nursing Home Market." *Inquiry* 17:25–41.

Scanlon, W. J. 1980. "Nursing Home Utilization Patterns: Implications for Policy." *Journal of Health Politics, Policy and Law* 4:619–41.

Schlenker, R. E., A. M. Kramer, P. A. Butler, J. A. Miller, R. G. Berg, & K. S. Bischoff. 1989. "Future Research on the Quality of Long-term Care Services in Community-based and Custodial Settings." Report for the Advisory Committee for "Research Synthesis and Recommendations on the Quality of Selected Long-term Care Services and on the Relationship between Long-term Care Services and Reduced Acute Care Expenditures." Center for Health Services Research, University of Colorado Health Sciences Center, Denver, Colo.

Shah, B. V., R. E. Folsom, F. E. Harrell, & C. N. Dillar. 1984. "Survey Data Analysis Software for Logistic Regression." Research Triangle, N.C.: Research Triangle Institute, November.

Shapiro, E., & R. B. Tate. 1985. "Predictors of Long-term Care Facility Use Among the Elderly." *Canadian Journal on Aging* 4:11–19.

Smits, H. L. 1984. "Incentives in Case-Mix Measures for Long-term Care." *Health Care Financing Review* 6(2).

Snider, E. 1980. "Awareness and Use of Health Services by the Elderly." *Medical Care* 18(12):1177–82.

Soldo, B. 1983. "In-Home Services for the Dependent Elderly: Determinants of Current Use and Implications for Future Demand." Urban Institute Publication Working Paper #1466–30, May.

Stoller, E. P. 1982. "Patterns of Physician Utilization by the Elderly: A Multivariate Analysis." *Medical Care* 20:1080–9.

Tessler, R., & D. Mechanic. 1975. "Consumer Satisfaction with Prepaid Group Practice: A Comparative Study." *Journal of Health and Social Behavior* 16:95–113.

U.S. Congress. Senate. Committee on Labor and Human Resources. 1988. A Bill to Amend the Public Health Service Act to Establish a Lifecare Long-term Care Program, and for other purposes. 100th Congress, Sess. 2, S.2681.

Von Behren, R. 1986. *Adult Day Care in America: Summary of a National Survey.* Washington, D.C.: National Institute for Adult Day Care of the National Council on Aging, Inc.

Wan, T. T. H., & B. Odell. 1980. "Factors Affecting the Use of Social and Health Services Among the Elderly." Paper presented to the American Public Health Association Annual Meeting, Detroit October 1980.

Wan, T. T. H., & S. Soifer. 1979. "A Multivariate Analysis of the Determinants of Physician Utilization." *Socio-Economic Planning Sciences* 9:229–37.

Ward, R. A. 1977. "Services for Older People: An Integrated Framework for Research." *Journal of Health and Social Behavior* 18:61–70.

Ware, J. E., A. Davies-Avery, and A. L. Stewart. 1978. "The Measurement and Meaning of Patient Satisfaction." *Health and Medical Care Services Review* 1:1.

Ware, J. E., M. K. Snyder, W. R. Wright, & A. R. Davies. 1983. "Defining and Measuring Patient Satisfaction with Medical Care." *Evaluation and Program Planning* 6:247–63.

Weiler, P. G., & E. Rathbone-McCuan. 1978. *Adult Day Care Community Work with the Elderly.* New York: Springer.

Weiler, P. G., P. Kim, & L. S. Pickard. 1976. "Health Care for Elderly Americans:

Evaluation of an Adult Day Health Care Model." *Medical Care* 14(8):700–708.

Weiss, G. L. 1988. "Patient Satisfaction with Primary Medical Care, Evaluation of Sociodemographic and Predispositional Factors." *Medical Care* 26(4):383–92.

Weissert, W. G. 1975. "Executive Summary." *Final Report: Adult Day Care in the U.S.: A Comparative Study.* Washington, D.C.: TransCentury Corporation.

Weissert, W. G. 1976. "Two Models of Geriatric Day Care: Findings from a Comparative Study." *Gerontologist* 16(5):420–27.

Weissert, W. G. 1977. "Adult Day Care Programs in the United States: Current Reserach Projects and a Survey of 10 Centers." *Public Health Reports* 92(1):49–56.

Weissert, W. G. 1978. "Costs of Adult Day Care: A Comparison to Nursing Homes." *Inquiry* 15(1):10–19.

Weissert, W. G., & C. M. Cready. 1989. "Toward a Model for Improved Targeting of Aged at Risk of Institutionalization." *Health Services Research* 24:4.

Weissert, W. G., C. M. Cready, & J. E. Pawelak. 1988. "The Past and Future of Home and Community-Based Long-Term Care." *Milbank Memorial Fund Quarterly* 66(2):309–88.

Weissert, W. G., T. Wan, B. Livieratos, & S. Katz. 1980. "Effects and Costs of Day Care Services for the Chronically Ill: A Randomized Experiment." *Medical Care* 18(6):567–84.

Wingard, D. L., D. W. Jones, & R. M. Kaplan. 1987. "Institutional Care Utilization by the Elderly: A Critical Review." *Gerontologist* 27:156–63.

Zastowny, T. R., K. J. Roghmann, & A. Hengst. 1983. "Satisfaction with Medical Care: Replications and Theoretic Reevaluation." *Medical Care* 21(3):294–318.

INDEX

Access to care, 46
Activities of daily living (ADL) dependencies: in DayCare software, 109; and full-time utilization, 32–33, 40; in Medicaid participants, 35–36; and participant satisfaction, 48, 49; prevalence of, 12; relation to models of care, 6, 7, 8, 11, 98
Aday, L. A., 44
Administrative costs, 85, 92
Admissions and discharge policies, 74, 76
Adult day care centers: activities at, 15; competition among, 37, 38, 40; conceptual model of, 3, 4, 105; cost-effectiveness of, 3; data sources on, 25; diagnostic correlates of use, 34; heterogeneity of, 9–10, 102; licenses of, 69–70; purposes of, 14–15; staffing levels, 80. *See also* Center-level variables; Models of care; Participant satisfaction; Services; Utilization
Adult Day Health Care Act (1978), 67
Age: country structure of, 38, 40; of day care participants, 12; and full-time utilization, 31, 40; relation to satisfaction with care, 44, 47, 57, 59, 100
Aldrich, J. H., 26
Allocated costs, 92
Alzheimer's disease, 33, 40, 79
American National Standards Institute (ANSI), 64
Andersen, R. M., 44
Area Agencies on Aging. *See* Older Americans Act
Area Resources File, 25
Auspice Model I, 97–98; effects on utilization of, 28–30, 31, 32, 33–34, 36, 37, 38, 41, 42, 99; expenses of, 79–80, 87, 90, 91, 92, 93, 95, 102; facilities and equipment, 18–19; funding levels, 82, 83, 84, 86, 88–89; funding sources, 19, 20, 35, 70, 71, 95, 101; licensure of, 70, 71; net income, 85–86; nonelderly participants, 117; participant characteristics, 11, 12–13, 21; and participant satisfaction, 55; percentage of utilization, 9, 10,

19; purposes of, 14–15; and satisfaction of caregivers, 60; services of, 15–17; staffing levels, 16, 18
Auspice Model II, 98; effects on utilization of, 31, 34, 36, 37, 38, 42, 98–99; expenses of, 79–80, 87, 90, 91, 92, 93, 95, 102; funding levels, 82, 83, 84–85, 86, 88–89; funding sources, 19, 20, 35, 70, 71, 95, 101; licensure of, 70, 71; net income, 85–86; nonelderly participants, 117; participant characteristics, 11, 12–13, 14, 21–22; and participant satisfaction, 55; percentage of utilization, 9, 10, 19; purposes of, 14–15; services of, 15–17, 22; staffing levels, 16, 18
Availability of services, 46

Bathing services, 72, 73
Benjamin, A. E., 24
Birnbaum, J., 67
Blind persons, day care centers for, 7, 9, 10
Bolda, E. J., 105
Branch, L. G., 24, 31, 32, 33
Brock, A. M., 24, 31

Cafferata, G. L., 24, 31
California: Department of Health Services, 68; licensing requirements in, 67–68; MediCal Assistance Program, 67, 68
Cancer: and full-time utilization, 34, 40; and satisfaction with day care, 51, 61
Capacity utilization, 93–94
Caregivers, informal, 14, 32; sampling of, 5; satisfaction with day care, 19, 59–61, 62–63, 100
Case management, 17, 72, 73
Case mix: in DayCare software, 109; measures of, and models of care, 6–7, 22
Center for Creative Living (Lexington, Ky.), 79, 80
Center operating capacity: and cost of care, 92–94, 96; and participant satisfaction, 39–40, 41, 96
Center-level variables: and caregiver satis-

Composed by Brushwood Graphics in Sabon
and Sabon bold text and display.

Printed by the Maple Press, Inc., on
Glatfelter's 60-lb. Hi-Brite Offset paper
and bound in Joanna Arrestox

Designed by Laury A. Egan